Unlocking the Mysteries of Death - New Perspectives for Post-mortem Examination

Edited by Kamil Hakan Dogan

Published in London, United Kingdom

Unlocking the Mysteries of Death - New Perspectives for Post-mortem Examination
http://dx.doi.org/10.5772/intechopen.1000429
Edited by Kamil Hakan Dogan

Contributors
Adis Salihbegović, Antonio Oliva, Carmen Cerda-Aguilar, Chitra Jangid, Cristina Basso, Edna Supur, Efe Jennifer Jaiyeoba-Ojigho, Elena Arbelo, Emina Dervišević, Eneko Barberia, Ermin Mašić, Estefanía Martínez-Barrios, Francesca Cazzato, Gaetano Thiene, George Sandusky, Georgia Sarquella-Brugada, Ishani Gupta, Jyoti Dalal, Lejla Dervišević, Lilian Ebele Chris-Ozoko, Lydia Emmert, María Luisa Ortega-Sánchez, Megan Szymanski, Melike Erbaş, Michael Yard, Muamer Dervišević, Muhamed Katica, Nina Čamdžić, Oscar Campuzano, Reetika Menia, Sahar Y. Issa, Sergio Cesar, Shivani Gandhi, Simone Grassi, Stefania Rizzo, Suada Kuskunović-Vlahovljak, Surbhi Mahajan, Vaishali Abrol, Vivian Valadares, William Aguilar-Navarro, Zurifa Ajanović

First published in London, United Kingdom, 2024 by IntechOpen
IntechOpen is the global imprint of INTECHOPEN LIMITED, registered in England and Wales, registration number: 11086078, 167-169 Great Portland Street, London, W1W 5PF, United Kingdom

British Library Cataloguing-in-Publication Data
A catalogue record for this book is available from the British Library

Additional hard and PDF copies can be obtained from orders@intechopen.com

Unlocking the Mysteries of Death - New Perspectives for Post-mortem Examination
Edited by Kamil Hakan Dogan
p. cm.
Print ISBN 978-1-83769-383-2
Online ISBN 978-1-83769-382-5
eBook (PDF) ISBN 978-1-83769-384-9

For EU product safety concerns:
IN TECH d.o.o., Prolaz Marije Krucifikse Kozulić 3, 51000 Rijeka, Croatia,
info@intechopen.com or visit our website at intechopen.com.

Meet the editor

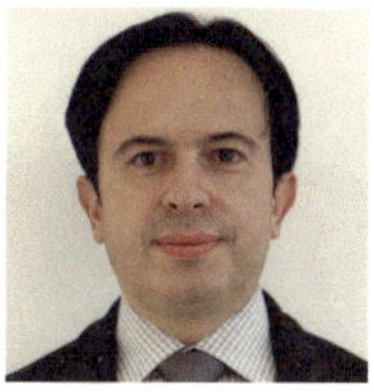

Kamil Hakan Dogan, MD, Ph.D., is a full professor and chair in the Department of Forensic Medicine, Selcuk University, Turkey. He received his MD from the Faculty of Medicine, Gazi University, Turkey, in 2000. After his extensive research in the forensic medicine field, he received his Ph.D. in Biochemistry in 2012. He gives lectures on forensic medicine and medical ethics to medical students as well as students in dentistry and law. He is the editor of five books and the *Bulletin of Legal Medicine* and a reviewer for several international journals. Dr. Dogan has published more than 200 articles in refereed journals, chapters in textbooks, and abstracts in scientific meetings.

Contents

Preface

Within investigations, forensic science acts as a guiding force, unraveling the mysteries of death and exposing the hidden truths within the remains of the deceased. Through this book *Unlocking the Mysteries of Death – New Perspectives for Post-mortem Examination*, readers will gain insight into innovative research and changing methods that inform our understanding of post-mortem investigations. It is with great pleasure that I introduce the assortment of chapters in this compilation, each playing a part in pushing the boundaries of forensic science.

Experts from diverse fields have come together in this book to offer their knowledge and perspectives on key elements of post-mortem examinations. The various chapters in this book cover a wide range of topics in forensic science, including molecular autopsies that uncover inherited arrhythmogenic diseases and the use of microbial communities to estimate post-mortem interval.

While moving forward in the chapters, we come across pioneering techniques like conducting limited genomic studies on rapidly collected post-mortem tissues and revitalizing decomposed and mummified tissues. The microbial witness, examined in a chapter delving into the unexplored potential of forensic microbiomes, introduces new approaches to understanding crime scenes and solving mysteries.

Forensic science is crucial for both criminal investigations and postmortem examinations, aiding in piecing together the complex stories behind the cause and manner of death and I believe that this book will provide readers with valuable insights into the recent progress in the field.

Kamil Hakan Dogan
Department of Forensic Medicine,
Selcuk University Faculty of Medicine,
Konya, Turkey

Chapter 1

Microbial Witness: Unraveling Mysteries with Forensic Microbiomes

Sahar Y. Issa

Abstract

Recent breakthroughs in forensic sciences, bioinformatics and next-generation sequencing technologies have broadened the application of microbiome analysis as an upcoming forensic tool. Studying the variation of the microbial flora and their profile, as well as the interactions among microorganisms, hosts, and the environment, are recent topics in microbiome research worldwide. Such novel microbiome applications have created a wide range of additional opportunities for the advancement of the forensic science. There are many modern forensic uses for the microbiome, such as postmortem identification, geolocation inference, and post-mortem interval prediction.

Keywords: microbiome, Forencic medicine, postmortem, identification, medicolegal, new advances, forensic microbiology, microbial forensics, microbial communities, Postmortem interval, high-throughput DNA sequencing, trace evidence, criminal investigations, ethical considerations

1. Introduction

In the context of forensics, the term "microbiome" refers to the collective community of microorganisms, including bacteria, fungi, viruses, and other microbes, that inhabit a specific environment or surface of interest, such as a crime scene, a victim's body, or evidence recovered from a crime scene [1]. These microorganisms leave behind unique traces and patterns, which forensic scientists can analyze and utilize to gain valuable insights and aid investigations. More Simply, The microbiome consists of all microorganisms and their DNA that inhabit a particular environment. Soils and oceans have distinct microbiomes, as do humans, animals, and vegetation [2].

Microbiomes in forensics can be found in various locations, including soil, skin, hair, and even on objects associated with a crime. By studying the composition and diversity of these microbial communities, forensic experts can potentially determine vital data that might help them in their daily work. These contributions include the time of death, postmortem interval, geographical origin, and other crucial information about a crime or incident [3]. Using microbiomes in forensics is an emerging field, offering a novel and promising approach to complement traditional forensic techniques and contribute to more accurate and comprehensive investigations [4].

Every crime scene contains microbes used as tangible evidence for over a century. Low-cost, high-throughput technologies enable the rapid accumulation of molecular data and the application of sophisticated machine-learning algorithms and artificial intelligence to develop criminal justice-relevant, generalizable predictive models. Integrating microbiome and metabolomic data has the potential to advance microbial forensics significantly [1, 5].

2. The microbiome analysis pathway

The microbiome analysis pathway involves several steps, from sample collection to data analysis. **Figure 1** is a basic outline of these critical stages. It's important to note that this is a simplified schema. However, the process can be more complex and involve additional steps depending on the specific case and available resources. Additionally, specialized training and expertise in microbiome analysis and forensic science are required to accurately perform and interpret the results.

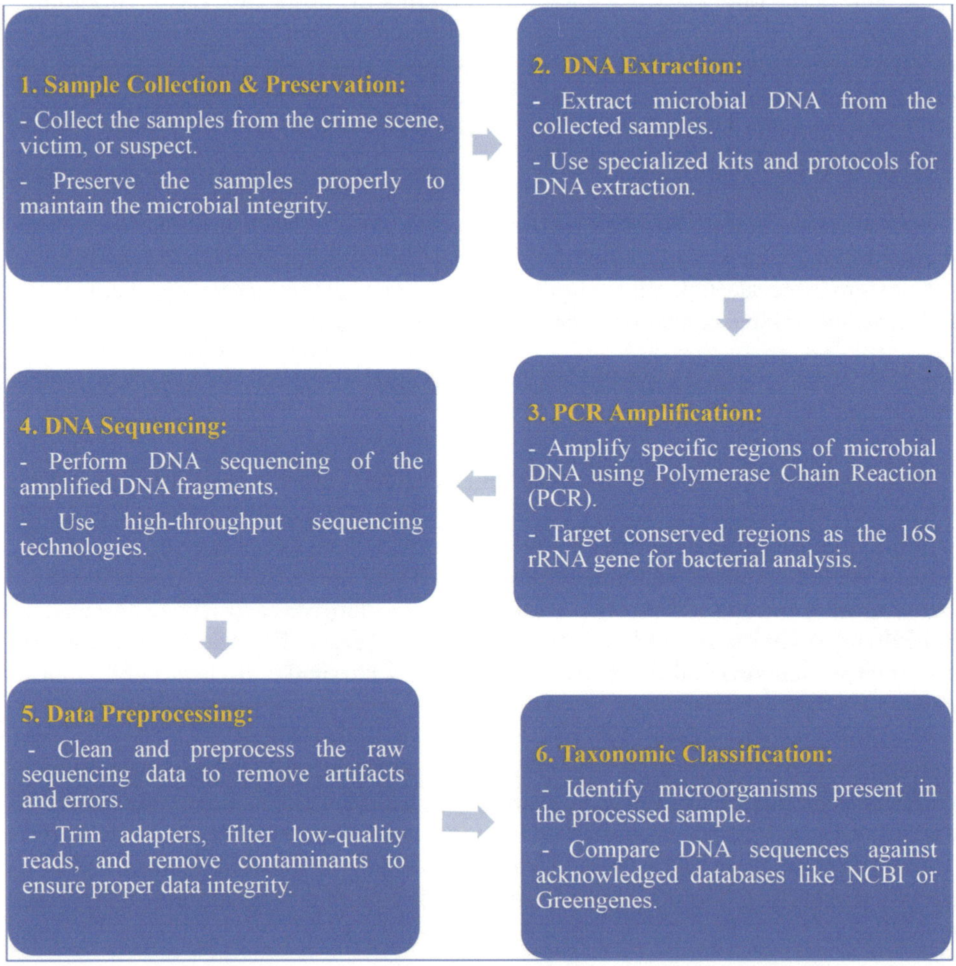

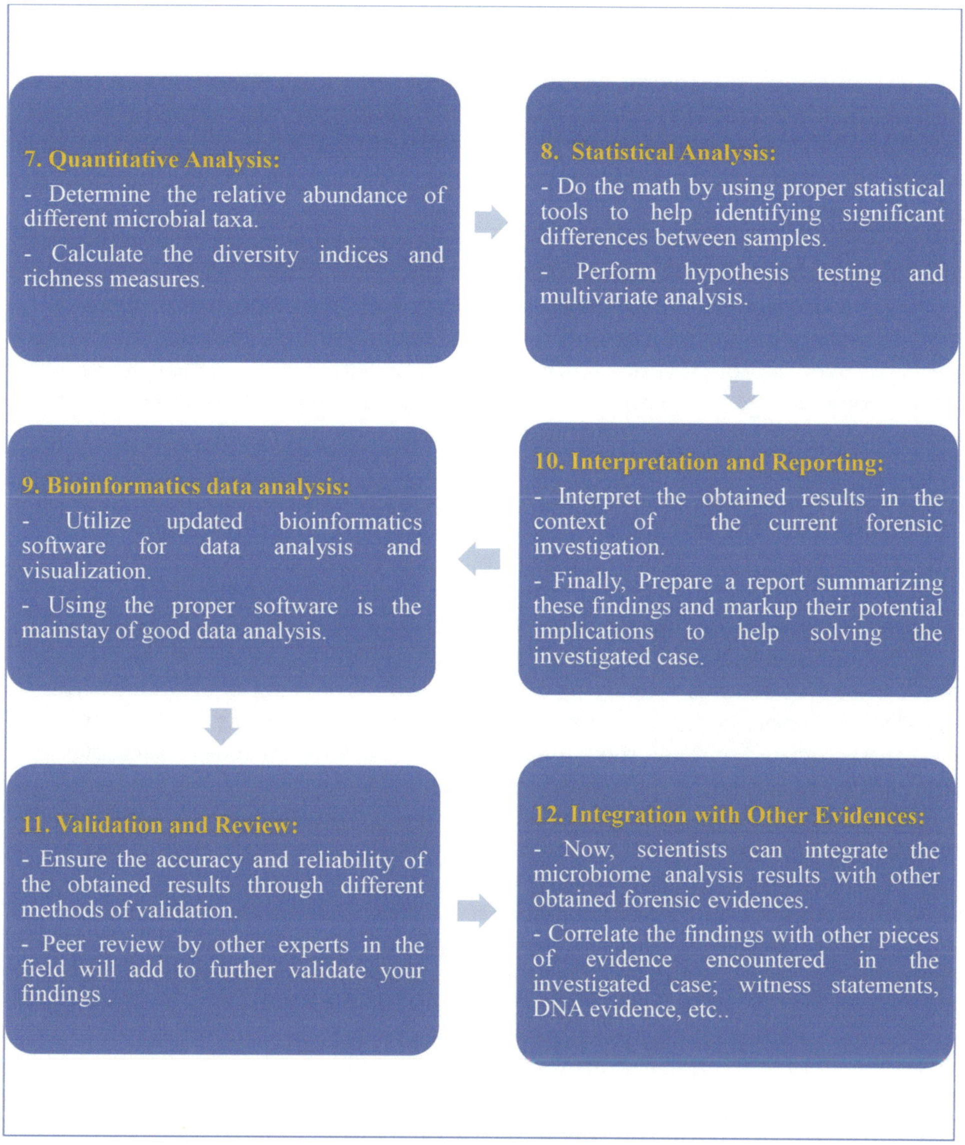

Figure 1.
A simplified schema summarizing the microbiome analysis pathway during forensic investigations.

3. Microbial forensics

Microbial Forensics is the term applied to the science of using microbiological techniques to analyze evidence for forensic attribution in situations spanning from bioterrorism to fraud, pathogen outbreaks, transmission, or the unintentional release of a biological agent or toxin. Biological and non-biological evidence are targeted for detection and characterization in microbial forensic investigations [6, 7].

Biological agents include microorganisms, protozoa, fungi, and toxins. Non-biological evidence, including additives, growth media, delivery devices, intelligence, etc. Biological and non-biological evidence can generate investigative leads and infer manufacturing and distribution processes [2, 8].

Forensic microbiomes in criminal investigations are expanding beyond biocrime, bioterrorism, and epidemiology. They are currently used to elucidate causes of death [such as drownings, toxicology, hospital-acquired infections, unanticipated child death, and shaken baby syndrome] and to aid in identifying mortals using microbiomes from the skin, hair, and body fluids. In addition, soil microbiomes assist in geolocation, while thanato-microbiome and epi-necrotic microbial communities are used to predict posthumous ages [9, 10]. Microbiomes are currently considered modern, reliable forensic investigation tools due to their current and prospective applications in various forensic investigations [3, 5].

The topic of microbiome forensics has been propelled by significant advancements in sequencing technology and computational pipelines, enabling the in-depth investigation of microbial communities with a high degree of species diversity. This methodology diverges from microbial forensics, which predominantly uses procedures tailored to detect and classify specific taxa of interest [11, 12].

4. The potential for microbial DNA as a source of trace evidence

Microbial forensics is a field that primarily concerns itself with the identification of certain strains of microorganisms linked to acts of terrorism, disease outbreaks, and instances of contamination. This discipline has extensively examined and investigated several strains for decades, employing a detailed analysis of genetic variations within individual genomes [13–15]. In contrast, the postmortem alterations and trace evidence signatures associated with microorganisms exhibit distinct variations in microbial communities, which can be most effectively analyzed using microbiome methodologies [16]. Numerous study groups have provided evidence of the potential of using microbiome data to estimate the postmortem interval (PMI), identify concealed burial sites, and establish connections between individuals and things or environments based on their skin microbiota [17–19]. The characteristics of microbial communities by employing advanced sequencing techniques were used to analyze gene markers that provide information about the evolutionary relationships or taxonomic classification (16S rRNA, 18S rRNA, and ITS). Additionally, statistical and computational methods, including machine learning, were utilized to analyze the data [1, 20].

5. Examples of microbiome forensic applications

Forensic microbiomes offer a growing capacity for microbial community identification and characterization, opening the door for microbial evidence in cases involving human identification, geolocation, and postmortem interval estimation, among other applications, as seen in **Figure 2**.

5.1 Postmortem interval estimation

Postmortem interval (PMI) estimation has always been an essential tool in forensic science. PMI has traditionally been estimated using physical, histomorphological, and biochemical techniques. However, preserving the forensic samples used in PMI estimation and surpassing the time limit for endogenous substance degradation largely compromise these traditional methods [21–23]. The organism undergoes irreversible physical and chemical changes after death. As time progresses, the accuracy of the current

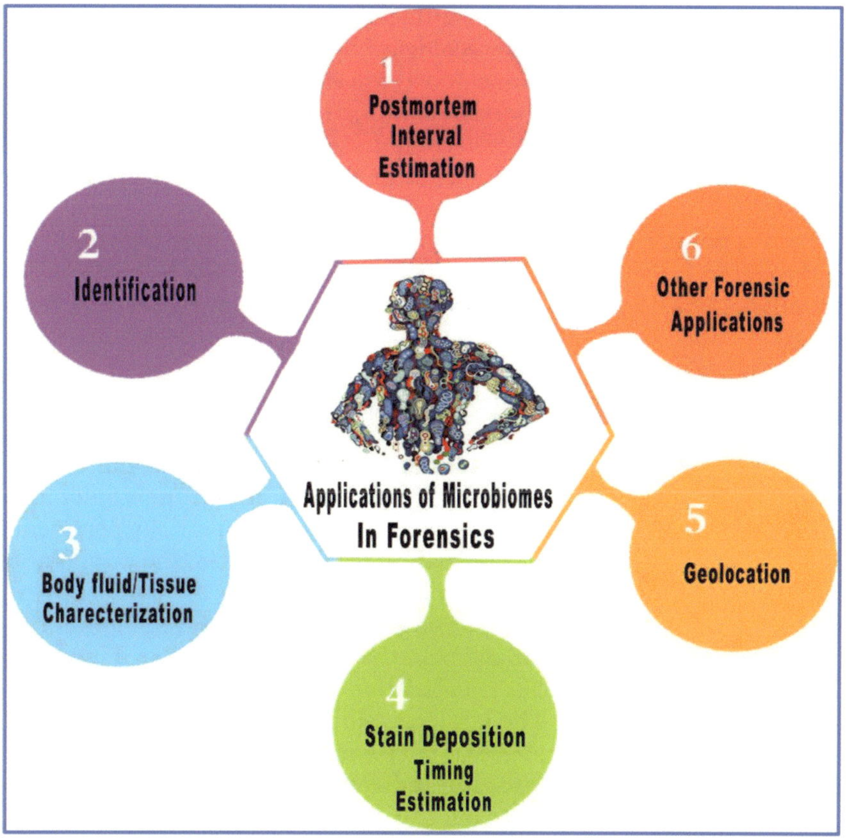

Figure 2.
Microbiome applications in forensic sciences.

methodologies for estimating PMI diminishes [24]. For decades, forensic entomology has been used to provide valuable estimates of time elapsed since death, but only if the death occurred between days and weeks ago. After this time limit, accuracy declines dramatically [25]. Here come the benefits of Metagenomics offering an alternative solution to this issue. Cadaver decomposes progressively after death due to the action of microorganisms. In the interim, tissue degradation products also progressively accumulate. As the duration of death increases, the quantity of spoilage microorganisms and products varies according to specific patterns. Therefore, the law of microbial community succession can be utilized to estimate PMI. Recently, the importance of metagenomic analysis in PMI estimation has grown [3, 8].

Different decay stages indicate the elapsed time since death, which can be calculated using changes in the variability and quantity of the microbiome in human corpses after death. However, it is essential to note that the bacterial succession that occurs at different stages of decomposition is influenced by physiological changes, fresh, bloated, active, and advanced decay, dry remains, and gender type. Each has diverse bacterial populations, which suggests the potential of microbiomes in criminal investigations to estimate the postmortem interval. In the future, it may be possible to investigate different microbiome communities in terms of decomposition to determine the actual time since death in addition to gender-specific microbiomes [7, 26].

Similar and repeatable microbiomes influence mammalian decomposition in various hosts and environments. This ecological hypothesis supports the PMI estimation method based on the microbiome. Most experiments have been conducted on animal models by obtaining postmortem samples from the abdomen, skin, scalp, and soil of experimental animals' cadaver decomposition systems. These studies yielded PMI estimates with a small mean absolute error. Scalp data yielded the lowest level of error [27].

The lack of a predictive model based on many human cadaver samples primarily restricts the method's application in forensic investigations. However, the potential for developing cadaveric microbiomes as a "clock" for estimating human PMI is immense [5].

5.2 Identification or individualization of unknown bodies

Individualization through skin microbiomes as a distinct and unique trait is a dream coming to reality through microbiome studies. A person's microbiome can be stable over time, making microbiome characterization potentially pertinent for forensic human identification. The human body's largest organ, the skin, is a complex living ecosystem supporting diverse microbial communities [14]. This helps establish the connection between human contact and evidence and that certain minor species are unique to particular individuals and have the capacity for personal recognition. Various substrates may facilitate the transmission of skin microbiome through direct or indirect skin-to-skin contact. The influence of individual microbial communities in public and private spaces revealed that microbiome variation is more significant between individuals than within the same individual [3].

5.3 Microbiomes in body fluid characterization

In contrast to body fluids like blood and semen, which are generally present in large quantities, traces of other fluids, such as vaginal fluid, urine, and sweat, have an essential role in DNA evidence. Identification is very obvious in forensic investigation cases of mixed body fluid, and it becomes a challenge to identify them separately [6, 9]. Microbial markers have been proposed as an alternative method of distinguishing between mixed body fluids. Each type of body fluid has a unique microbial makeup that can be used as bio-indicators, with the microbial composition inferring the kind of body fluid present. Different body fluids carry different types of bacteria that can be identified in this way. For instance, vaginal discharge often contains *Lactobacillus crispatus*, *Lactobacillus jensenii*, and *Atopobium vaginae*. Saliva often contains *Streptococcus salivarius* and *Streptococcus mutans* [28].

Particularly in the cases of an alleged sexual assault, microbial communities' identification will undoubtedly be beneficial, whereby the spatial placement of such biological samples can fix sexual relationships and support the testimony of victims or suspects [11].

5.4 Stain deposition time estimation

The time estimation since the deposition of a stain at a crime scene can be a valuable tool for law enforcement to evaluate the alibis of identified suspects and witnesses and generate investigative leads to determine the appropriate perpetrator [14].

Until recently, the forensic application of studying microbial composition in a microbiome setting has not been thoroughly explored. However, new research has demonstrated that DNA and RNA analysis can identify time-dependent changes in the microbial composition of human biological traces [12, 17]. Estimating the time elapsed since an individual's salivary stain deposition, for example, can be primarily achieved using DNA profiling of commensal bacteria. This method exhibits an average error rate of 5 days when applied within the initial 30-day period following the deposition of the stain. Nevertheless, additional investigation is required to gain a more comprehensive understanding and provide a more accurate representation of the microbial alterations pertaining to this application [27].

5.5 Geolocation during crime scene investigations

The human microbiome can be influenced by various circumstances, some of which may serve as a means to deduce the geographical origin of a host through the examination of microbiome samples obtained from human evidence found at crime scenes. The criteria encompassed in this analysis comprise geographical latitude, industrialization in the country of residency, and cultural and societal components [25].

Microbial community composition of things belonging to individuals residing within the same geographical places has more similarity to those of the individuals living in different areas. Human microbiome analysis has the potential to determine the city of origin for human biological samples accurately. Identifying the geographic sources of unidentified cadavers was facilitated by the appearance of *Helicobacter pylori* strains in the context of forensic casework. In the event of a satisfactory outcome, integrating microbiome-based geolocation analysis and bio-geographic ancestry [BGA] research utilizing human ancestry informative DNA markers will yield supplementary geographic data about the individual being examined [18].

5.6 Other forensic science applications of microbiomes

Microbiome analysis in forensic medicine encompasses other various applications, including ethnicity and possible living conditions, determining the cause of death, such as drowning, cardiovascular-related fatalities, and deaths associated with drug usage. In addition, the genotyping of microorganisms related to sexually transmitted illnesses can serve as a valuable tool for identifying the primary source of infection, a factor of particular significance within the legal and law enforcement domains [29]. In some instances, establishing a connection between the infectious microbe present in the suspect, the source of infection, and the victim, the infected individual, has been found beneficial. This approach has been valuable in identifying the perpetrator of child abuse [15].

Metagenomic research of microbial communities can yield insights about an individual's racial and ethnic background. For example, individuals residing in economically disadvantaged rural regions who have not been exposed to commercial antibiotics exhibit more bacterial diversity and enhanced functionality in their skin than those utilizing alternative therapeutic antibiotics [7]. Nonetheless, variations in the composition of the human microbiome among different ethnic groups are influenced to some extent by factors such as dietary patterns, lifestyle choices, and geographical surroundings [12].

6. The challenges and ethical perspectives surrounding forensic microbiome analysis

The utilization of metagenomics in the field of forensics is now in its nascent stages. The utilization of microbiomes as a shred of exclusive evidence for individual identity, geolocation inference, and postmortem interval [PMI] estimates has not yet received official approval. There is a lack of established operational principles and requirements for microbiological evidence extraction, packaging, transportation, and preservation. Furthermore, there is a pressing need to enhance the trustworthiness of microbiome tools utilized in forensics. Further validation is necessary to establish the specificity and stability of individual microorganisms in comparison to human DNA markers [30].

Further investigation is needed to enhance our understanding of the microbiome's trustworthiness in the context of forensic applications and to establish error rates that can be deemed trustworthy. To effectively tackle the issue at hand, it is imperative to employ a sample size of considerable magnitude and utilize quantitative machine learning methodologies [18]. Various well-established methods, such as K-nearest neighbor models, random forest models, and neural networks, have been extensively used in forensic applications involving the microbiome, namely in the domains of classification and regression [4]. Machine learning techniques have demonstrated a clear benefit in effectively handling multidimensional datasets, particularly in the context of microbiome data. However, it is necessary to do the quantitative computation of pertinent forensic factors. There exist notable disparities between the existing evaluation techniques employed in elucidating microbiome evidence and the conventional likelihood calculation utilized for human DNA [21]. Additional study is required for the evaluation criteria to gain acceptance within the forensic scientific community [8].

However, it is imperative to have a sample size that is large enough for machine learning techniques to achieve satisfactory performance. Hence, it is essential to create microbiome databases to employ their proper use in forensic science effectively. Implementing forensic DNA databases has facilitated law enforcement agencies in identifying or eliminating individuals connected to criminal activities [24]. Furthermore, this technological advancement enabled the identification of serial criminals through the correlation of several cases, enhancing forensic evidence's evidentiary significance [19]. The application of microbiomes as a forensic tool has been hindered by the fragmented condition of publically available databases despite the sequential creation of several microbiome databases, such as the Human Microbiome Project [HMP] and Earth Microbiome Project [EMP]. Using 16S rRNA gene sequencing data obtained from publically accessible sources can facilitate the identification and characterization of the Forensic Microbiome Database [FMD], enabling the derivation of insights about its original location of discovery. There is a growing demand for more databases to cater to diverse forensic applications [31]. Ultimately, the establishment of awareness is a crucial component in rendering forensic science admissible. The cost of training and acquiring equipment for sequencing microbiomes is substantial. The reduction in prices will be facilitated by advancements in sequencing technology and increased computational capabilities. The aforementioned concerns hold significant importance in forensic microbiomes and are expected to be resolved with the advancement of related scientific research. In addition to its previous uses, metagenomics has the potential to yield significant improvements in forensic pathology, toxicology, and drug addiction testing. In summary, integrating metagenomics into forensics can offer novel insights and resolutions for forensic identification [32].

Author details

Sahar Y. Issa
Department of Forensic Medicine and Clinical Toxicology, Faculty of Medicine, Alexandria University, Egypt

*Address all correspondence to: sahar.issa@alexmed.edu.eg

References

[1] Braga RM, Dourado MN, Araujo WL. Microbial interactions: Ecology in a molecular perspective. Brazilian Journal of Microbiology. 2016;**47**:86-98. DOI: 10.1016/j. bjm.2016.10.005

[2] Giampaoli S, Alessandrini F, Frajese GV, et al. Environmental microbiology: Perspectives for legal and occupational medicine. Legal Medicine. 2018;**35**:34-43. DOI: 10.1016/j.legalmed.2018.09.014

[3] Huttenhower C, Gevers D, Knight R, et al. Structure, function, and diversity of the healthy human microbiome. Nature. 2012;**486**:201-214. DOI: 10.1038/ nature11234

[4] Oliveira M, Amorim A. Microbial forensics: New breakthroughs and future prospects. Applied Microbiology and Biotechnology. Dec 2018;**102**(24):10377-10391. DOI: 10.1007/s00253-018-9414-6. Epub 2018 Oct 9. PMID: 30302518; PMCID: PMC7080133

[5] Neckovic A, Van Oorschot RAH, Szkuta B, et al. Investigation of direct and indirect transfer of microbiomes between individuals. Forensic Science International Genetics. 2020;**45**:102212. DOI: 10.1016/j.fsigen.2019.102212

[6] Park J, Kim SJ, Lee JA, et al. Microbial forensic analysis of human-associated bacteria inhabiting hand surface. Forensic Science International: Genetic Supplement Series. 2017;**6**:510-512. DOI: 10.1016/j.fsigss.2017.09.210

[7] Kakizaki E, Kozawa S, Matsuda H, et al. Freshwater bacterioplankton cultured from liver, kidney, and lungs of a decomposed cadaver retrieved from a sandy seashore: Possibility of drowning in a river and then floating out to sea. Legal Medicine. 2010;**12**(4):195-199. DOI: 10.1016/j. legalmed.2010.03.008

[8] Lopez CD, Vidaki A, Ralf A, et al. Novel taxonomy-independent deep learning microbiome approach allows for accurate classification of different forensically relevant human epithelial materials. Forensic Science International Genetics. 2019;**41**:72-82. DOI: 10.1016/j. fsigen.2019.03.015

[9] Lopez CD, Gonzalez DM, Haas C, et al. Microbiomebased body site of origin classification of forensically relevant blood traces. Forensic Science International Genetics. 2020;**47**:102280. DOI: 10.1016/j.fsigen.2020

[10] Tackmann J, Arora N, Schmidt TSB, et al. Ecologically informed microbial biomarkers and accurate classification of mixed and unmixed samples in an extensive cross-study of human body sites. Microbiome. 2018;**6**:192. DOI: 10.1186/s40168-018-0565-6

[11] Escapa LF, Chen T, Huang Y. New insights into human nostril microbiome from the expanded Human Oral Microbiome Database (eHOMD): A resource for the microbiome of the human aerodigestive tract. mSystems. 2018;**3**. DOI: e00187, 10.1128/ mSystems.00187-18

[12] Ritari J, Salojarvi J, Lahti L, et al. Improved taxonomic assignment of human intestinal 16S rRNA sequences by a dedicated reference database. BMC Genomics. 2015;**16**:1-10. DOI: 10.1186/ s12864-015-2265-y

[13] Marcelino R, Holmes V, Sorrell EC. The use of taxon-specific reference databases compromises

metagenomic classification. BMC Genomics. 2020;**21**:184. DOI: 10.1186/s12864-020-6592-2

[14] Dobay A, Haas C, Fucile G, et al. Microbiome-based body fluid identification of samples exposed to indoor conditions. Forensic Science International Genetics. 2019;**40**:105-113. DOI: 10.1016/j.fsigen.2019.02.010

[15] Zhang R, Walker AR, Datta S. Unraveling city-specific signature and identifying sample origin locations for the data from CAMDA MetaSUB challenge. Biology Direct. 2021;**16**:1. DOI: 10.1186/s13062-020-00284-1

[16] The Human Microbiome Project Consortium. A framework for human microbiome research. Nature. 2012;**486**:215-221. DOI: 10.1038/nature11209

[17] Ehrlich SD, The MetaHIT Consortium. MetaHIT: The European Union Project on metagenomics of the human intestinal tract. In: Nelson K, editor. Metagenomics of the Human Body. New York, NY: Springer; 2011. pp. 307-316. DOI: 10.1007/978-1-4419-7089-3_15

[18] Yang J, Tsukimi T, Yoshikawa M, et al. Cutibacterium acnes (*Propionibacterium acnes*) 16S rRNA genotyping of microbial samples from possessions contributes to owner identification. mSystems. 2019;**4**:e00594-19. DOI: 10.1128/mSystems.00594-19

[19] Belk A, Xu ZZ, Carter DO, et al. Microbiome data accurately predicts the postmortem interval using random forest regression models. Genes. 2018;**9**:104. DOI: 10.3390/genes9020104

[20] Blekhman R, Goodrich JK, Huang K, et al. Host genetic variation impacts microbiome composition across human body sites. Genome Biology. 2015;**16**:191-196. DOI: 10.1186/s13059-015-0759-1

[21] Dominianni C, Sinha R, Goedert JJ, et al. Sex, body mass index, and dietary fiber intake influence the human gut microbiome. PLoS One. 2015;**10**:e0124599. DOI: 10.1371/journal.pone.0124599

[22] Fettweis JM, Brooks JP, Serrano MG, et al. Differences in vaginal microbiome in African American women versus women of European ancestry. Microbiology. 2014;**160**:2272-2282. DOI: 10.1099/mic.0.081034-0

[23] Monda V, Villano I, Messina A, et al. Exercise modifies the gut microbiota with positive health effects. Oxidative Medicine and Cellular Longevity. 2017;**2017**:3831972-3831978. DOI: 10.1155/2017/3831972

[24] Tridico SR, Murray DC, Addison J, et al. Metagenomic analyses of bacteria on human hairs: A qualitative assessment for applications in forensic science. Investment Genetics. 2014;**5**:16. DOI: 10.1186/s13323- 014-0016-5

[25] Javan GT, Finley SJ, Can I, et al. Human thanatomicrobiome succession and time since death. Scientific Reports. 2016;**6**:29598. DOI: 10.1038/srep29598

[26] Can I, Javan GT, Pozhitkov AE, et al. Distinctive thanatomicrobiome signatures found in the blood and internal organs of humans. Journal of Microbiological Methods. 2014;**106**:1-7. DOI: 10.1016/j.mimet.2014.07.026

[27] Damann FE, Williams DE, Layton AC. Potential use of bacterial community succession in decaying human bone for estimating postmortem interval. Journal of Forensic Sciences. 2015;**60**:844-850. DOI: 10.1111/1556-4029.12744

[28] Hauther KA, Cobaugh KL, Jantz LM, et al. Estimating time since death from postmortem human gut microbial communities. Journal of Forensic Sciences. 2015;**60**:1234-1240. DOI: 10.1111/1556-4029.12828

[29] Johnson HR, Trinidad DD, Guzman S, et al. A machine learning approach for using the postmortem skin microbiome to estimate the postmortem interval. PLoS One. 2016;**11**:e0167370. DOI: 10.1371/journal.pone.0167370

[30] Hyde ER, Haarmann DP, Petrosino JF, et al. Initial insights into bacterial succession during human decomposition. International Journal of Legal Medicine. 2015;**129**:661-671. DOI: 10.1007/s00414-014-1128-4

[31] Donaldson AE, Taylor MC, Cordiner SJ, et al. Using oral microbial DNA analysis to identify expirated bloodspatter. International Journal of Legal Medicine. 2010;**124**:569-576. DOI: 10.1007/s00414-010-0426-8

[32] Power DA, Cordiner SJ, Kieser JA, et al. PCR-based detection of salivary bacteria as a marker of expirated blood. Science & Justice. 2010;**50**:59-63. DOI: 10.1016/j.scijus.2009.04.006

Chapter 2

Exploring the Potential of Microbial Communities: Understanding Their Role in PMI Estimation

Chitra Jangid and Jyoti Dalal

Abstract

Cadaver decomposition is a natural phenomenon intimately affected by numerous organisms such as insects, bacteria etc., where they use the decaying body as their nutrition source. These organisms can be utilized in forensic science to estimate the Post-mortem Interval. Forensic entomology is one of the popular approaches where successive colonization of insects on cadaver is studied to estimate PMI. However, sometime this method does not provide consistent results due to lack of insect activities during cold environment conditions or when crime scene is indoor. Recently, researchers have noted that microbiomes have shown predictable and clockwise successional patterns on decomposing cadavers and suggested this could be utilized to estimate PMI when this approach is etched with other established methods. This chapter summarizes the utility of microbial profiling in medico-legal investigations.

Keywords: post-mortem interval (PMI), microbial communities, cadaver, decomposition, succession pattern

1. Introduction

In forensic investigations, PMI estimation is crucial, especially when the exact time of death is uncertain or in doubt. It acts as a crucial criterion to estimate the sequence of events leading to the person's death, supporting the reconstruction of the incident's conditions, and making it easier to identify prospective suspects [1]. As it helps law enforcement authorities gather evidence, establish alibis, and link suspects to the crime scene, a precise measurement of PMI is crucial for criminal investigations [2]. Additionally, by ensuring that justice is done, and the rights of the deceased are maintained, estimating PMI contributes to preserving the overall accuracy and integrity of the legal system. Rigor mortis, the stiffening of muscles after death, has been used as an indicator of PMI. It usually starts shortly after death, peaks between 12 and 24 hours later, and then slowly fades away [3]. However, the onset and duration of rigor mortis might vary depending on conditions including temperature and physical activity [4]. Another common technique for estimating PMI is livor mortis, or the settling of blood in the dependent areas of the body. Forensic examiners can calculate the PMI and establish the location of the body after death by examining the color and dispersion of the livor mortis [5]. Algor mortis, the cooling of the body, has also been utilized for PMI estimation [5]. By measuring the temperature of the body and the ambient environment, forensic investigators can estimate the time since death [5]. Few authors have applied total body scoring method based on the appearance of three separate regions, the head, trunk, and limbs for estimating PMI. Megyesi et al. [6] developed this method for estimating PMI using accumulated day degree (ADD) degree days in human remains. Later, this method was later modified by Heaton et al. [7] to estimate Post-mortem submersion interval (PMSI) in human remains. Although the rate of decomposition is highly variable and affected by factors such as temperature, humidity, and insect activity, it might be difficult to estimate the accurate PMI using only the stages of decomposition. The assessment of PMI has also been done using chemical changes in the body, such as potassium levels in the vitreous humor and hypostasis patterns [8]. The necessity for more sophisticated and precise procedures in PMI assessment is highlighted by the fact that each of these old methods has its own drawbacks, including subjectivity, variability, and the influence of outside influences [1, 9]. Since conventional methods for PMI assessment in forensic investigations have substantial limitations, alternative strategies are being investigated. Microbial forensics, which uses the power of microbial communities present on and within the deceased individual, is a new area with significant potential for PMI estimate. Microbial forensics investigates the composition, diversity, and microbial activity related to the decomposition process in order to calculate the PMI [10–12]. This strategy acknowledges that microbial communities exhibit diverse patterns of succession through time and are crucial to the breakdown process [2]. Researchers may be able to create more precise and dependable approaches for PMI estimation by studying these microbial alterations. Numerous research has shown how useful microbiological forensics may be for PMI estimate. As an example, researchers have explored microbial composition of diverse body regions, including the skin, oral cavity, and gastrointestinal system, and have discovered distinct microbial succession patterns linked to various stages of decomposition. Researchers have been able to identify certain microbial signatures that correlate with the PMI by using high-throughput sequencing methods and bioinformatic studies [2, 13–15]. These discoveries open the door to the establishment of databases and forensic technologies based on microorganisms that can help investigators to determine the time since death more precisely.

Although decomposition in aquatic environments has received less study, it is not a rare occurrence in investigations, with a primary focus on detecting the presence of diatoms, algae, and scavenging activity of aquatic species [16–18]. Only a few authors have discussed the utility of microbial communities in estimating PMI [16, 19, 20]. In a study conducted by Cartozzo et al. [20], they estimated PMI in freshwater by studying the successional pattern and associated changes in the bacterial community within submerged skeletal remains of pigs. The microbial communities were identified using 16S rRNA sequencing, revealing the presence of phyla such as *Firmicutes*, *Proteobacteria*, *Acidobacteria*, *Bacteroidetes*, and *Spirochaetes*. Collectively, these studies suggest that PMI can be predicted by observing the repeatability of microbial community succession during decomposition.

2. Stages of decomposition

Decomposition is a continuous process which begins with the changes at the cellular level. The degradation process continues even when the bones reach to dry remains stage until the whole nutrients get into to the natural ecosystem and thus energy is recycled.

Goff [5] described five stages of decomposition in his study which are discussed below.

1. Fresh Stage: The fresh phase starts as soon as the death occurs and remains until bloating occurs. Apart from the deposition of eggs by flies in the natural cavities such as nose, eyes, ears and the areas of tissue dehiscence, this phase does not exhibit any insect activity. Blowflies and flesh flies are the earliest flies to reach the cadaver.

2. Bloated Stage: Putrefaction occurs during this phase of decomposition. Putrefaction is a process of tissue decay by the action of microbes that are generally associated with the gut of the deceased [21, 22]. During this process, gases such as ammonia, hydrogen sulphide, and methane are released inside the body, leading to a balloon-like appearance of the corpse [23, 24]. The temperature also rises due to the combined effect of putrefaction and the metabolic activities of fly maggots. Flies and their larvae are most abundant during this phase. Seepage of fluid from natural orifices, when it mixes with the ammonia gas, deteriorates the soil fauna and increases the pH of the soil.

3. Decay Stage: The decay stage begins with the rupture of the skin, enabling gases to escape and the collapse of the abdominal cavity. Extensive maggot infestation can be observed during this phase. As part of faunal succession, flies are eventually replaced by beetles [24, 25]. Necrophagous and predatory taxa are seen in significant numbers in the later stages of the decay stage, whereas certain predatory taxa, including Staphylinidae species, were present during the bloated stage. The majority of Calliphoridae and Sarcophagidae will have completed pupariation by the end of this stage and left the remains. By the time the decay stage is complete, dipteran larvae will have mostly removed the flesh from the remains.

4. Post-decay Stage: The corpse in this stage reduces to skin, cartilage, and bone. Flies are no longer dominant. The number of species and individuals of Coleoptera increases. These species feed on the dried flesh and cartilage from the bones, giving them a clean appearance.

5. Skeletal Stage: During this stage, only bones and hair remain. Most of the arthropods are absent, or if present, they are in very few numbers [25]. The area beneath the remains gradually returns to its usual soil fauna.

3. Microbial communities and decomposition

Microbial forensics makes use of the fact that the human body contains a diverse array of microbial communities known as the human microbiome. These microbial communities play significant roles in many physiological processes and have the ability to persist and evolve reliably after death [26]. They also help with the release of gases like methane and hydrogen sulphide as well as volatile compounds that give decomposition its distinctive odor [3]. These microbial communities also help break down organic matter into simpler forms that may be utilized by other organisms, which contributes to the recycling of nutrients [8]. Diversity and composition of decomposition-related microbial communities vary depending on a number of factors, including the location of the body, the environment, and the individual. Microbial communities that exhibit different patterns of microbial succession can be observed on the skin [27], oral cavity [28, 29], gastrointestinal tract [30–32], and other regions of the body that are vulnerable to decomposition. Thanks to advancements in molecular biology technologies like high-throughput DNA sequencing, the study of microbial communities in human decomposition has undergone a radical transformation. By studying the DNA or RNA retrieved from postmortem samples, researchers can identify and define the microbial species present and learn more about the specific microorganisms involved in the decomposition process.

4. Succession of microbial communities and building microbial clock

Studying microbial communities in human decomposition for forensic investigations has a number of benefits. It can assist with more accurate PMI estimation, for example, by analyzing the pattern of microbial succession and the presence of specific microorganisms connected to distinct breakdown phases. Studies have shown that microbial communities undergo predictable changes over time with the progress in decomposition process, allowing for the construction of a timeline for PMI estimation [12–15, 19, 33]. Although much progress has been made in the recognition of microbial community contribution during decomposition, there are still many unknowns. Sample handling practices, DNA extraction techniques, and data processing practices must all be standardized for research to be comparable and reproducible. Additionally, it is crucial to consider and control the effects of outside elements including the environment and sample processing.

Microbial forensics considers functional changes in microbial communities after decomposition in addition to taxonomic variations. Researchers have conducted studies to characterize the microbial succession and establish a microbial clock for PMI estimation [2, 33]. By sampling the microbial communities present on a decomposing body and analyzing their composition and abundance, forensic scientists can compare the microbial profile to reference data collected from known PMI cases. This comparison allows them to estimate the time since death based on the similarities and differences in microbial succession. In 2014, Pechal et al. [26] developed a framework shown in **Figure 1** to estimate post mortem interval from bacterial community. In real-world forensic investigations, this paradigm offered a conceptual roadmap for combining microbiological succession data into the computation of PMI. Their research identified seven families (*Fusobacteriaceae*, *Clostridiales Incertae Sedis XI*, *Aerococcaceae*, *Micrococcaceae*, *Campylobacteraceae*, *Comamonadaceae*, *Moraxellaceae*, *Bacteroidetes*) and four phyla (*Proteobacteria*, *Actinobacteria*, *Firmicutes*) as potentially significant predictors of estimating physiological. Additionally, the use of statistical models and machine learning techniques has improved the precision and dependability of PMI calculation utilizing microbial forensics. Predictive models can be created to estimate PMI with more precision by incorporating several parameters, such as

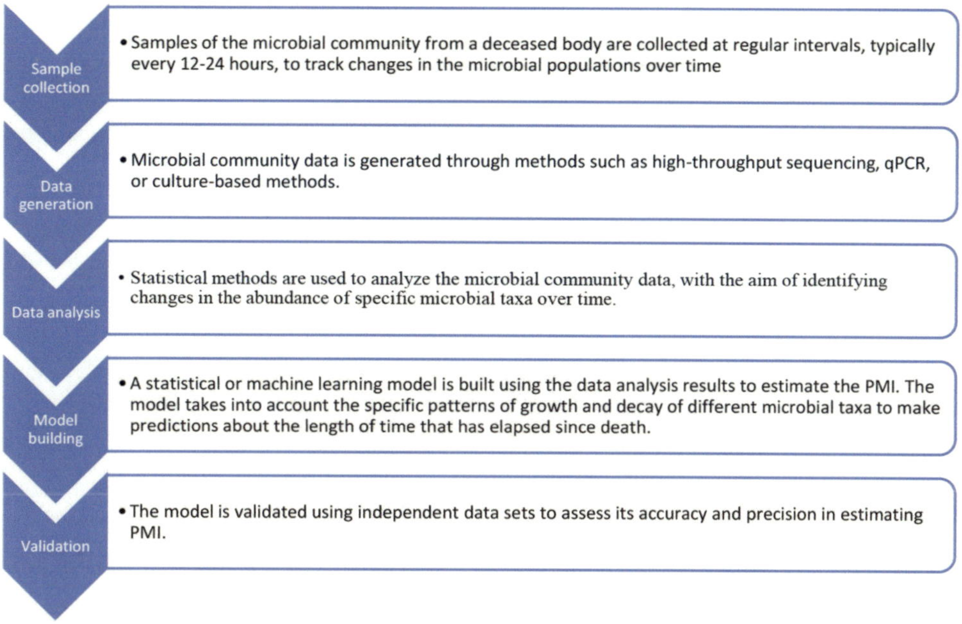

Figure 1.
Framework to estimate post mortem interval from bacterial community [26].

taxonomic abundance, functional profiles, environmental conditions, and weather data [14, 27, 28, 34–36]. As additional information about the dynamics of microbial communities during decomposition is produced and included in the study, these models keep becoming better. Although microbiological forensics has a lot of potential as a method for PMI estimate, there are a number of obstacles and restrictions that need to be overcome.

5. Investigating the temporal changes in microbial communities during decomposition

Microbial postmortem interval (PMI) assessment must take into account the temporal changes in microbial populations during decomposition. Researchers can improve PMI estimation techniques and obtain important insights into the breakdown process by examining the dynamic changes in microbial populations over time. This field has used a variety of technologies, including culture-dependent and culture-independent techniques, as well as advanced molecular biology methods including DNA sequencing, metagenomics, and metabolomics.

A basic strategy for comprehending the temporal dynamics of microbial communities during decomposition is time-series sampling. In order to characterize microbial populations at various phases of decomposition, samples must be taken at various points after death [37]. Researchers can pinpoint temporal patterns and changes connected to various PMI phases by tracking the composition, variety, and abundance of microbes over time [10, 38, 39]. Shotgun metagenomics and 16S rRNA gene sequencing are two examples of high-throughput sequencing methods that have revolutionized the study of microbial communities during decomposition. These techniques allow for the identification, measurement, and evaluation of the functional potential

References	specimen	Microbial findings	Estimated PMI
[47]	Blood, brain, heart, liver and spleen	*Clostridium sp*. in heart, liver, spleen and *Lactobacillus* in blood were prominent bacterial species observed.	20-240 h PMI
[48]	Intestine, oral cavity and skin	Aerobic to anaerobic bacterial shift was noted. *Firmicutes, Actinobacteria* and *Bacteroidetes* were prominent.	0–30 days decomposition
[49]	Pericardial fluid, portal vein liver, mesenteric lymph node and blood	*Escherichia sp., Enterococcus sp., Staphylococcus sp.* and *Clostridium* were prominent.	1–7 days
[34]	Lower rib	*Chloroflexi, Acidobacteria Firmicutes, Actinobacteria, Proteobacteria* and *Bacteroides,* were prominent phyla found.	571–18,918 ADD decomposition
[31]	Proximal large intestine	*Bacteroides* and *Lactobacillus* declining abundance was noted to estimate PMI.	9–20 days decomposition
[45]	heart, spleen, liver, buccal cavity, blood and Brain	Higher abundance of *Pseudomonas* and *Clostridials* were found in Female cadavers while male cadavers have higher abundance of *Clostridium, Clostridiales*, and Streptococcus as decomposition progress.	3.5–240 h PMI
[28]	Oral cavity	*Firmicutes* and *Actinobacteria* were found prominent during decomposition.	0–12 days decomposition
[30]	Proximal large intestine (caecum)	Significant decline in *Bacteroidetes* while increase in *Clostridiales* and *Gammaproteobacteria, Ignatzschineria* and *Wohlfahrtiimonas* was noted.	0–800 ADD decomposition
[50]	Liver and spleen tissues	Post-mortem Clostridium Effect was observed.	4-78 h PMI
[14]	Rectum, nares, eyes, mouth, umbilicus and external auditory canal,	Decline in *Actinobacteria* and *Bacteroidetes* with increase in abundance of *Proteobacteria* was observed as decomposition progresses.	1–73 + h PMI
[51]	transverse colon and the vermiform appendix	*Firmicutes, Bacteroidetes*, and their respective subclasses	5-192 h PMI
[52]	Skin	most abundant families were *Moraxellaceae, Burkholderiaceae (Proteobacteria),* and *Clostridiaceae (Firmicutes),*	0–7415 + accumulated degree hours (ADH)
[53]	A cloacal swab, large intestine, ceca, and Small intestine,	*Lactococcus, Serratia*, and *Clostridium*	0-72 h PMI
[54]	Oral cavities	*Atopostipes*, *Fack lamia* and *Ceras bacillus* were linearly correlated at all 12 time points in the 59-day period.	0–59 days decomposition

Table 1.
Association of prominent microbial taxa with different decomposition stages of different animal models.

of various microbial species [40, 41]. Researchers can determine how the relative abundance of different taxa has changed over time by analyzing the sequencing data derived from time-series samples [10, 38, 39]. To establish links between microbial dynamics and the breakdown process, these results can be connected with PMI. Another effective approach for examining the temporal variations in microbial activity during decomposition is metabolomics, the study of small-molecule metabolites. Understanding microbial communities' metabolic processes can be accomplished by examining the volatile organic compounds (VOCs) and other metabolites they create [24]. Researchers can better understand the metabolic activities of various microbial species during decomposition and their relationship to PMI by analyzing the temporal patterns of these metabolites. Another method used to comprehend the metabolic capability of microbial communities during decomposition is functional profiling. Researchers can uncover the functional genes and pathways involved in organic matter decomposition, nutrient cycling, and other pertinent processes by using metagenomic or metatranscriptomic techniques [41, 42]. The activity and functional changes of microbial communities over time can be learned from the temporal examination of functional profiles, which helps with PMI calculation.

Large-scale microbiological datasets created from time-series samples can be analyzed using bioinformatics and statistical analysis. The processing, quality control, taxonomic assignment, and functional annotation of microbial sequencing data are made easier by data analysis pipelines like QIIME, Mothur, and MG-RAST [43]. In order to find relevant temporal trends, microbiological markers, and create PMI prediction models, statistical approaches like multivariate analysis, linear regression, and machine learning algorithms are also used [10, 27, 44, 45]. The temporal changes in microbial communities during decomposition have been investigated using these methods in several research. In a time-series investigation on decomposing human remains, for instance, Metcalf et al. [2] found distinct changes in the microbial communities throughout time, with particular species predominating during various phases of decomposition. Dekeirsschieter et al. [46] conducted research on the volatile organic chemicals released during decomposition and isolated particular molecules linked to various stages of decomposition. **Table 1** represent the association of prominent microbial taxa with animal models with different decomposition stages.

6. Factors influencing the composition and succession of microbial communities during decomposition

Numerous elements that affect the dynamics of microbial colonization and activity have an impact on the composition and succession of microbial communities during decomposition. Accurately evaluating the microbial profiles linked to breakdown processes requires an understanding of these parameters. Environmental circumstances, corpse location, and interspecies interactions are only a few of the variables that might affect the composition and succession of microbial communities during postmortem decomposition [15]. The composition of microbial communities during postmortem decomposition is greatly influenced by environmental factors, including temperature, moisture content, soil type, soil texture and oxygen availability [55, 56]. The rate and course of decomposition are significantly influenced by temperature. According to Carter et al. [56], high temperatures hasten tissue breakdown by accelerating microbial activity and low temperatures slow down degradation and lower microbial community activity. The amount of moisture is also important since it influences the water availability required for microbial growth and enzymatic activity [56]. Areas with high moisture content may be more conducive to microbial colonization and breakdown [55, 56]. On the other hand, oxygen availability affects the kinds of microbial communities that are present during decomposition. In oxygen-rich environments, aerobic decomposition favors the growth of aerobic bacteria and fungi, whereas anaerobic decomposition favors the activity of anaerobic microbial groups, such as sulfate-reducing bacteria [48]. The composition of the microbial community during postmortem decomposition is also influenced by the body's location. Different bodily sites have different environmental characteristics, such as temperature, moisture content, and oxygen levels, which affect microbial colonization and succession in different ways. In contrast, buried bodies may experience lower temperatures and lower oxygen levels, which would favor the activity of anaerobic microbial communities [57]. For instance, exposed body surfaces may experience higher temperatures and increased oxygen availability, favoring the growth of aerobic microorganisms. Additionally, the presence of nearby soil or water may introduce new microbial species, changing the makeup of the community [57].

Interspecies interactions are important in determining the dynamics of the microbial community during postmortem decomposition. Microbes interact in a variety of ways, including competition, collaboration, and predation, which can have an impact on the composition and succession of communities. Microbial species may become dominated by some groups and excluded by others due to competition for resources [40]. By facilitating the breakdown of complex organic molecules, cooperative interactions like cross-feeding and syntrophy can improve the efficiency of decomposition. Necrophagous insects and scavengers can also influence microbial communities by modifying the availability of nutrients and spreading microbes across various body regions [45]. The diversity of microbes is also significantly shaped by maggot activity throughout the decomposition stages. Maggots actively feed on decomposing organic matter as the larvae of flies, which has a significant effect on microbial dynamics. The mechanical disruption caused by their eating and movement of the decaying material increases the surface area available for microbial colonization and speeds up the decomposition of organic materials [56]. According to Pechal et al. [40], certain microbial groups can be inhibited or selected for by medications, embalming fluids, and other chemical agents, changing the breakdown process. The dynamics of the microbial community can also be impacted using antibiotics during life or the presence of naturally occurring antimicrobial substances in body tissues, which may change the rate of breakdown and the types of organisms involved [58].

7. Advancement in techniques employed in microbial PMI estimation

In order to estimate the time since death, microbiological PMI estimates entails examining the changes in microbial communities linked to decomposing remains. To investigate microbial composition, diversity, and functional activity during decomposition, numerous methods and procedures have been developed. Utilizing molecular biology tools like DNA sequencing, metagenomics, and metabolomics, these techniques cover both culture-dependent and culture-independent procedures. Advancements in microbial identification techniques have significantly contributed to our understanding of postmortem microbial communities and their implications in forensic investigations. One widely used technique is 16S rRNA gene sequencing, which targets the highly conserved region of the 16S rRNA gene to identify and classify bacterial and archaeal taxa. This approach provides valuable information about the composition and diversity of microbial communities associated with decomposition processes [59]. The development of high-throughput sequencing platforms, such as Illumina and Ion Torrent, has greatly enhanced the efficiency and speed of 16S rRNA gene sequencing, enabling comprehensive characterization of microbial communities present on decomposing cadavers [4].

Another advanced technique is metagenomic shotgun sequencing, which involves the sequencing of all the DNA present in a microbial sample, including both the microbial and host DNA [60]. This method offers deeper understanding of the microbial community, allowing for the identification of not only bacteria but also viruses, fungi, and other microorganisms. Metagenomic shotgun sequencing has been instrumental in revealing the functional potential of microbial communities during decomposition, providing insights into metabolic activities and pathways associated with postmortem processes [48]. Advancements in bioinformatics tools and databases have also played a crucial role in microbial identification. The development of specialized databases, such as the Ribosomal Database Project (RDP) and the Greengenes database, has facilitated accurate taxonomic assignment of microbial sequences obtained through high-throughput sequencing [33]. Additionally, advanced bioinformatics pipelines and algorithms have been developed to process large-scale sequencing data and perform taxonomic profiling, allowing for more accurate identification and characterization of microbial communities [61].

Other techniques, such as quantitative polymerase chain reaction (qPCR), have also seen advancements in the context of postmortem microbial identification. qPCR enables the quantification of specific microbial taxa by targeting conserved regions of their genomes. This technique has been used to assess the relative abundance of certain bacterial species associated with decomposition, providing quantitative data that can be used in estimating PMI [13]. The application of NGS technologies in postmortem microbial community analysis has provided valuable insights into the temporal dynamics of microbial succession during decomposition. By analyzing the changes in microbial composition over time, researchers have identified specific microbial taxa associated with different stages of decomposition. For example, studies have shown that certain bacteria, such as members of the genera Clostridium and Bacteroides, are more abundant during the advanced stages of decomposition when anaerobic conditions prevail. Moreover, NGS technologies have enabled the detection of low-abundance microorganisms that may have important forensic implications. These technologies are highly sensitive and can detect microbial taxa present in minute quantities. This sensitivity is crucial when dealing with postmortem samples where the microbial biomass may be low or unevenly distributed across different body sites. In addition to microbial identification, NGS technologies have facilitated the analysis of microbial functional potential. Metagenomic sequencing allows researchers to predict the functional capabilities of microbial communities based on the presence of specific genes or functional pathways. This information can provide insights into the metabolic activities of microbial communities during decomposition and their potential roles in various stages of PMI estimation. The use of NGS technologies for the identification and analysis of microbial communities associated with postmortem processes has significantly advanced the field of forensic microbiology. These technologies have provided a more comprehensive understanding of the complex microbial dynamics during decomposition, offering potential applications for estimating PMI more accurately.

8. Microbial communities presence at different body organs

Approximately 1–10 trillion microbes, including bacteria, archaea, and fungi, reside inside the human body. Prior to birth, the human body is free from any type of microbes, but after birth, a complex microflora develops as these microorganisms begin to colonize, and this colonization continues throughout life. Each individual has a unique microbial composition that undergoes various changes and fluctuations depending on factors such as lifestyle, genetics, and food intake [62]. The earlier belief of internal organs being sterile was challenged by the Human Microbiome Project (HMP) [63]. Although the abundance of microorganisms varies from one organ to another, the composition of the microbiome differs between bodily regions due to site-specific conditions. The HMP studied the microbiome of seven body sites, including the nasal passage, skin, gut, oral cavity, and urogenital region, in healthy individuals [63]. The prominent bacterial phyla differed among these sites, with Firmicutes and Bacteroidetes being most abundant in the gut, Actinobacteria, Firmicutes, and Proteobacteria being prominent on the skin, and Fusobacteria, Bacteroidetes, Firmicutes, and Proteobacteria being prominent in the oral cavity. During decomposition, the richness of microbial communities increases, but overall diversity decreases, meaning that the number of individuals of species decreases [30]. This decrease in diversity may be due to varying abilities of microbial species to respond to the environment, with some species able to reproduce while others may fail [30]. Microbes associated with the decomposition process have been the subject of numerous investigations [28]. These studies have explored microbial communities in different locations of the body, such as the skin, gut region, internal organs, and oral cavities. Several of these studies will be discussed in the following section.

1. Skin: The largest organ in the human body, the skin, is essential in defending against microbial invasion. The epidermis, however, becomes more permeable as a result of the breakdown process, allowing microorganisms to colonize and aid in the decomposition process. According to studies, the skin displays various microbial successions as it decomposes [45]. Metcalf et al. [2] examined mice carcass skin as well as grave soil and found association of *Gammaproteobacteria* in both cases. In addition, the association of the family *Pseudomonadaceae* was also found dominant over the mouse skin. However, considerable quantities of *Moraxellaceae* bacteria have been found associated with the skin of a swine carcass during the first 24 hours of decomposition by Pechal et al. [26] and the number decreases as the decomposition progresses.

2. Oral Cavity: Different microbial communities related to the human host can be found in the nasal and oral cavities. These microbial communities are important in these regions' tissues' degradation during decomposition. The Oral cavity contains around 1000 types of microbial taxa from phyla such as *Aponeurophytes*, *Proteobacteria*, *Synergists*, *Firmicutes*, *Actinomycetes* and *Bacteroidetes* [64]. The relative abundance of *Actinobacteria* was found decreasing with rise in PMI, which is similar to findings of other previous microbial studies of oral cavity in decomposing [28, 36]. Adserias-Garriga et al. [28] also described the successional changes in the oral cavity microbes in decomposing cadaver from early putrefaction stage to the skeletonized stage.

3. Gut: A complex microbial community that supports overall health and plays a critical role in nutrition metabolism is found in the gut. The release of nutrients from the disintegrating tissues causes the gut microbial community to undergo major alterations throughout decomposition. Gut region is mostly dominated by *Bacteroidetes* and *Firmicutes* with smaller populations of *Proteobacteria* and *Actinobacteria*. Several studies have investigated the microbial communities of gut region, especially from caecum region. For example, microbial communities from gut region of 12 human cadavers were evaluated in a study conducted by Hauther et al. [31] where three bacterial genera were quantified by qPCR and target gene was 16S rRNA. The relative abundance of *Bacteroides* and *Lactobacillus* were found to be decreasing exponentially with increase in PMI and was suggested that these microbial species could be used as quantitative indicators of PMI. Later, DeBruyn & Hauther [30] observed evident change in microbial species with PMI where decline in *Bacteroidetes* and increase in *Clostridial* (*Clostridium, Anaerosphaera*) and *Gamma proteobacteria* (*Ignatzschineria* and *Wohlfahrtiimonas*) was noted. These microbes help transform complex molecules into simpler ones, such as proteins and carbohydrates. Numerous volatile organic compounds (VOCs) are produced by the metabolic processes of gut bacteria and can be employed as PMI indicators.

4. Viscera: During decomposition, the internal organs, also referred to as viscera, support various microbial communities. While the external microbial taxa are involved in the skin decomposition, internal organs usually remain free from microbial species interaction in healthy individuals [15]. However, after the death of the individual, the immune system of body does not work and microbial community present in the gut region of the individual starts spreading to the other organs [15]. Microbes overpower the immune system and enters into the internal organs within the 24 hours of the death [65]. The rate of decomposition does vary from one organ to another depending on its role in biological activity. Among all the internal organs, microbial communities of brain, liver, spleen and heart have stable composition. The uterus or prostate, for instance, normally decays last and lack enzymatic activity, while the putrefaction in the gut and intestine starts within a few hours [66]. Burcham et al. [42] tracked translocation of *Staphylococcus* and *Clostridium perfringens* in internal organs during decomposition using whole body fluorescent imaging and culture-based techniques. Structural and functional changes in the microbial taxa during decomposition of caecum, heart, bone marrow and lungs were observed in Rat carcass. The observation of this study co-related to several other study of microbial communities during decomposition such as [36, 50, 67].

5. Other: Several studies have been conducted to explore the microbial communities of burial cadavers. Decomposing environment of burial cadaver are quite different than the cadavers decomposing in the exposed environment. Thus, the microbial communities of these cadavers may be different than the other bodies due to different temperature, oxygen availability, humidity etc., Receiving the cadavers which have been buried in the grave is not so rare in the Forensic legal medicine investigations. Procopio et al. [68] studied successional pattern of soil microbial community in buried pig carcasses using metabarcoding approach where 16SrRNA gene (Variable region 4) was sequenced. They observed

significant increase in *Firmicutes*, *Proteobacteria*, and *Bacteroidetes* at specific PMIs as well as a decrease in *Acidobacteria*. Additionally, along with the change in composition of microbial communities on surface and internal organs of the cadaver, change in microbial communities of soil around the decomposition cadaver also occur. Cobaugh et al. [41], observed such changes in the microbiome of surrounding soil of human cadavers. Study conducted by Metcalf et al. [67] revealed that microbial diversity of soil surrounding cadaver is generalized across selective season, ecosystem and microbial taxa of host and exchange of microbial species between the host and the surround soil may occur.

9. Future direction and limitations

The use of microbial communities to estimate postmortem interval (PMI) holds great promise for forensic investigations. However, there are several future directions and limitations that need to be addressed to enhance the reliability and applicability of this approach. One future direction is the integration of multi-omics approaches in studying postmortem microbial communities. This involves combining metagenomic sequencing with other "-omics" techniques such as metatranscriptomics, metaproteomics, and metabolomics. By incorporating these approaches, researchers can obtain a more comprehensive understanding of the functional activities and interactions within postmortem microbial communities. This integration can provide valuable insights into the specific metabolic processes and molecular mechanisms involved in decomposition, which can further improve the accuracy of PMI estimation. Another important aspect for future development is the establishment of standardized protocols and databases specific to postmortem microbial analysis. Standardization of sample collection, processing, and analysis methods is crucial to ensure reproducibility and comparability of results across different studies. Additionally, the creation of comprehensive and curated databases that catalog microbial taxa associated with decomposition and their temporal dynamics would greatly facilitate microbial identification and analysis. These databases could serve as valuable references for PMI estimation, enabling the comparison of microbial community profiles in different postmortem scenarios.

Despite the potential of using microbial communities for PMI estimation, there are limitations that should be addressed. One limitation is the influence of external factors on microbial communities, such as environmental conditions and the presence of scavengers or competing microorganisms. These factors can introduce variability in microbial succession patterns and make it challenging to establish universal correlations between microbial profiles and PMI [1]. Therefore, future research should focus on understanding and accounting for the impact of these external factors on postmortem microbial communities to improve the accuracy of PMI estimation. Another limitation is the lack of comprehensive longitudinal studies that monitor microbial succession from the time of death to advanced decomposition stages. Long-term studies that track microbial communities over extended periods will provide valuable insights into the temporal dynamics of microbial succession and the stability of microbial profiles for PMI estimation [26]. Such studies would allow for the development of more accurate models and algorithms that incorporate the complex interplay between microbial communities and decomposition processes. The future direction of using microbial communities for PMI estimation lies in integrating multi-omics approaches, establishing standardized protocols and databases, and conducting comprehensive longitudinal studies. Overcoming the limitations associated with external factors and the lack of long-term studies will be essential in further improving the accuracy and reliability of microbial-based PMI estimation, ultimately enhancing the capabilities of forensic investigations.

10. Conclusion

Despite its promise, microbial forensics in PMI estimation is still a developing field with several challenges to overcome. Standardization of methods, protocols, and data analysis techniques is necessary to ensure reproducibility and comparability of results across different studies and forensic laboratories [1]. Additionally, the influence of confounding factors, such as environmental conditions, the presence of personal care products, and variations in microbial communities among individuals, needs to be thoroughly investigated and accounted for [2]. Ethical considerations, including sample collection procedures and privacy concerns, should also be addressed to ensure responsible and ethical application of microbial forensics in PMI estimation. In conclusion, microbial forensics is an emerging field that shows great potential in PMI estimation. By harnessing the power of microbial communities associated with the decomposition process, researchers can gain valuable insights into the postmortem interval. However, further research is needed to validate these findings across different environmental contexts and refine the predictive models. The continued exploration of microbial succession patterns and their correlation with PMI holds great promise in enhancing forensic investigations and providing valuable information for the justice system.

Conflict of interest

Author declares no conflict of interest.

Author details

Chitra Jangid and Jyoti Dalal*
Department of Forensic Science, Lovely Professional University, Punjab, India

*Address all correspondence to: jyotidalal417@gmail.com

References

[1] Carter DO. The importance of microbial communities in the estimation of the time since death. In: Estimation of the Time since Death. London, United Kingdom: Elsevier; 2020. pp. 109-139. DOI: 10.1016/b978-0-12-815731-2.00006-6

[2] Metcalf JL, Wegener Parfrey L, Gonzalez A, Lauber CL, Knights D, Ackermann G, et al. A microbial clock provides an accurate estimate of the postmortem interval in a mouse model system. eLife. 2013;**2**:1-19. DOI: 10.7554/elife.01104

[3] Carter DO, Yellowlees D, Tibbett M. Cadaver decomposition in terrestrial ecosystems. Naturwissenschaften. 2007;**94**:12-24. DOI: 10.1007/s00114-006-0159-1

[4] Clarke TH, Gomez A, Singh H, Nelson KE, Brinkac LM. Integrating the microbiome as a resource in the forensics toolkit. Forensic Science International. Genetics. 2017;**30**:141-147. DOI: 10.1016/J.FSIGEN.2017.06.008

[5] Goff ML. Early postmortem changes and stages of decomposition. In: Current Concepts in Forensic Entomology. Netherlands: Springer; 2010. pp. 1-24. DOI: 10.1007/978-1-4020-9684-6_1

[6] Megyesi MS, Nawrocki SP, Haskell NH. Using accumulated degree-days to estimate the postmortem interval from decomposed human remains. Journal of Forensic Sciences. 2005;**50**:1-9. DOI: 10.1520/JFS2004017

[7] Heaton V, Lagden A, Moffatt C, Simmons T. Predicting the postmortem submersion interval for human remains recovered from U.K. waterways. Journal of Forensic Sciences. 2010;**55**:302-307. DOI: 10.1111/j.1556-4029.2009.01291.x

[8] Jarvis H, Marc O. Estimation of the Time since Death: Current Research and Future Trends. London, United Kingdom: Academic Press; 2020

[9] Madea B. Is there recent progress in the estimation of the postmortem interval by means of thanatochemistry? Forensic Science International. 2005;**151**:139-149. DOI: 10.1016/J.FORSCIINT.2005.01.013

[10] Metcalf JL. Estimating the postmortem interval using microbes: Knowledge gaps and a path to technology adoption. Forensic Science International. Genetics. 2019;**38**:211-218. DOI: 10.1016/j.fsigen.2018.11.004

[11] Cai J, Guo Y, Zha L, Guo J. The role of the microbiome in PMI estimation. In: Forensic Ecogenomics: The Application of Microbial Ecology Analyses in Forensic Contexts. Tess valley, United Kingdom: Elsevier; 2018. pp. 113-131. DOI: 10.1016/B978-0-12-809360-3.00005-9

[12] Dash HR, Das S. Thanatomicrobiome and epinecrotic community signatures for estimation of post-mortem time interval in human cadaver. Applied Microbiology and Biotechnology. 2020;**104**:9497-9512. DOI: 10.1007/s00253-020-10922-3

[13] Benbow ME, Pechal JL, Lang JM, Erb R, Wallace JR. The potential of high-throughput metagenomic sequencing of aquatic bacterial communities to estimate the postmortem submersion interval. Journal of Forensic Sciences. 2015;**60**:1500-1510. DOI: 10.1111/1556-4029.12859

[14] Pechal JL, Schmidt CJ, Jordan HR, Benbow ME. A large-scale survey of the postmortem human microbiome, and its potential to provide insight into

the living health condition. Scientific Reports. 2018;**8**:1-15. DOI: 10.1038/s41598-018-23989-w

[15] Javan GT, Finley SJ, Abidin Z, Mulle JG. The thanatomicrobiome: A missing piece of the microbial puzzle of death. Frontiers in Microbiology. 2016;7:225. DOI: 10.3389/FMICB.2016.00225/BIBTEX

[16] Dickson GC, Poulter RTM, Maas EW, Probert PK, Kieser JA. Marine bacterial succession as a potential indicator of postmortem submersion interval. Forensic Science International. 2011;**209**:1-10. DOI: 10.1016/j.forsciint.2010.10.016

[17] Haefner JN, Wallace JR, Merritt RW. Pig decomposition in lotic aquatic systems: The potential use of algal growth in establishing a postmortem submersion interval (PMSI). Journal of Forensic Sciences. 2004;**49**:330-336

[18] Zimmerman KA, Wallace JR. The potential to determine a postmortem submersion interval based on algal/diatom diversity on decomposing mammalian carcasses in brackish ponds in Delaware. Journal of Forensic Sciences. 2008;**53**:935-941. DOI: 10.1111/J.1556-4029.2008.00748.X

[19] Kaszubinski SF, Receveur JP, Nestle Bsc ED, Pechal JL, Benbow ME. Microbial community succession of submerged bones in an aquatic habitat. Journal of Forensic Science. 2022;**67**:1565-1578. DOI: 10.1111/1556-4029.15036

[20] Cartozzo C, Simmons T, Swall J, Singh B. Postmortem submersion interval (PMSI) estimation from the microbiome of Sus scrofa bone in a freshwater river. Forensic Science International. 2021;**318**:110480. DOI: 10.1016/j.forsciint.2020.110480

[21] Paczkowski S, Schütz S. Post-mortem volatiles of vertebrate tissue. Applied Microbiology and Biotechnology. 2011;**91**:917-935. DOI: 10.1007/S00253-011-3417-X

[22] Dent BB, Forbes SL, Stuart BH. Review of human decomposition processes in soil. Environmental Geology. 2004;**45**:576-585. DOI: 10.1007/S00254-003-0913-Z

[23] Gennard D. Forensic Entomology: An Introduction. Chichester, UK: John Wiley & sons; 2007

[24] Vass AA. Review of: Soil analysis in forensic Taphonomy: Chemical and biological effects of buried human remains. Journal of Forensic Sciences. 2008;**53**:1484-1485. DOI: 10.1111/j.1556-4029.2008.00886.x

[25] Ahmad NW, Lim LH, Dhang CC, Chin HC, Abdullah AG, Mustaffa WNW, et al. Comparative insect fauna succession on indoor and outdoor monkey carrions in a semi-forested area in Malaysia. Asian Pacific Journal of Tropical Biomedicine. 2011;**1**:S232-S238. DOI: 10.1016/S2221-1691(11)60161-5

[26] Pechal JL, Crippen TL, Benbow ME, Tarone AM, Dowd S, Tomberlin JK. The potential use of bacterial community succession in forensics as described by high throughput metagenomic sequencing. International Journal of Legal Medicine. 2014;**128**:193-205. DOI: 10.1007/s00414-013-0872-1

[27] Johnson HR, Trinidad DD, Guzman S, Khan Z, Parziale JV, DeBruyn JM, et al. A machine learning approach for using the postmortem skin microbiome to estimate the postmortem interval. PLoS One. 2016;**11**:1-23. DOI: 10.1371/journal.pone.0167370

[28] Adserias-Garriga J, Quijada NM, Hernandez M, Rodríguez Lázaro D, Steadman D, Garcia-Gil LJ. Dynamics of the oral microbiota as a tool to estimate time since death. Molecular Oral Microbiology. 2017;**32**(6):511-516. DOI: 10.1111/omi.12191

[29] Dong K, Xin Y, Cao F, Huang Z, Sun J, Peng M, et al. Succession of oral microbiota community as a tool to estimate postmortem interval. Scientific Reports. 2019;**9**:13063. DOI: 10.1038/s41598-019-49338-z

[30] DeBruyn JM, Hauther KA. Postmortem succession of gut microbial communities in deceased human subjects. PeerJ. 2017;**5**:e3437. DOI: 10.7717/PEERJ.3437

[31] Hauther KA, Cobaugh KL, Jantz LM, Sparer TE, Debruyn JM. Estimating time since death from postmortem human gut microbial communities. Journal of Forensic Sciences. 2015;**60**:1234-1240. DOI: 10.1111/1556-4029.12828

[32] Martínez Aragonés ÁA, Martínez-Manzanares E, Tapia-Paniagua ST. Early post mortem interval estimation in a mouse model using molecular analyses of the gut thanatomicrobiome. Spanish Journal of Legal Medicine. 2022;**48**:107-114. DOI: 10.1016/J.REMLE.2022.02.002

[33] Finley SJ, Benbow ME, Javan GT. Microbial communities associated with human decomposition and their potential use as postmortem clocks. International Journal of Legal Medicine. 2015;**129**:623-632. DOI: 10.1007/s00414-014-1059-0

[34] Damann FE, Williams DE, Layton AC. Potential use of bacterial community succession in decaying human bone for estimating postmortem interval. Journal of Forensic Sciences. 2015;**60**:844-850. DOI: 10.1111/1556-4029.12744

[35] Palazzo C, Pelletti G, Fais P, Giorgetti A, Boscolo-Berto R, Gaudio RM, et al. Application of aquatic decomposition scores for the determination of the post mortem submersion interval on human bodies recovered from the northern Adriatic Sea. Forensic Science International. 2021;**318**:110599. DOI: 10.1016/j.forsciint.2020.110599

[36] Guo J, Fu X, Liao H, Hu Z, Long L, Yan W, et al. Potential use of bacterial community succession for estimating post-mortem interval as revealed by high-throughput sequencing. Scientific Reports. 2016;**6**:24197. DOI: 10.1038/srep24197

[37] Hyde ER, Haarmann DP, Petrosino JF, Lynne AM, Bucheli SR. Initial insights into bacterial succession during human decomposition. International Journal of Legal Medicine. 2014;**129**:661-671. DOI: 10.1007/s00414-014-1128-4

[38] Liu R, Wang Q, Zhang K, Wu H, Wang G, Cai W, et al. Analysis of postmortem intestinal microbiota successional patterns with application in postmortem interval estimation. Microbial Ecology. 2021;**84**(4):1087-1102. DOI: 10.1007/s00248-021-01923-4

[39] Deel H, Bucheli S, Belk A, Ogden S, Lynne A, Carter DO, et al. Using microbiome tools for estimating the postmortem interval. In: Microbial Forensics. London, United Kingdom: Elsevier; 2019. pp. 171-191. DOI: 10.1016/B978-0-12-815379-6.00012-X

[40] Pechal JL, Crippen TL, Tarone AM, Lewis AJ, Tomberlin JK, Benbow ME. Microbial community functional change during vertebrate carrion decomposition.

PLoS One. 2013;**8**:1-11. DOI: 10.1371/journal.pone.0079035

[41] Cobaugh KL, Schaeffer SM, DeBruyn JM. Functional and structural succession of soil microbial communities below decomposing human cadavers. PLoS One. 2015;**10**:1-20. DOI: 10.1371/journal.pone.0130201

[42] Burcham ZM, Pechal JL, Schmidt CJ, Bose JL, Rosch JW, Eric Benbow M, et al. Bacterial community succession, transmigration, and differential gene transcription in a controlled vertebrate decomposition model. Frontiers in Microbiology. 2019;**10**:745. DOI: 10.3389/FMICB.2019.00745/BIBTEX

[43] D'Argenio V, Casaburi G, Precone V, Salvatore F. Comparative metagenomic analysis of human gut microbiome composition using two different bioinformatic pipelines. BioMed Research International. 2014;**2014**:325340. DOI: 10.1155/2014/325340

[44] Belk A, Xu ZZ, Carter DO, Lynne A, Bucheli S, Knight R, et al. Microbiome data accurately predicts the postmortem interval using random Forest regression models. Genes (Basel). 2018;**9**:104. DOI: 10.3390/GENES9020104

[45] Javan GT, Finley SJ, Can I, Wilkinson JE, Hanson JD, Tarone AM. Human thanatomicrobiome succession and time since death. Scientific Reports. 2016;**6**:29598. DOI: 10.1038/srep29598

[46] Dekeirsschieter J, Verheggen FJ, Gohy M, Hubrecht F, Bourguignon L, Lognay G, et al. Cadaveric volatile organic compounds released by decaying pig carcasses (Sus domesticus L.) in different biotopes. Forensic Science International. 2009;**189**:46-53. DOI: 10.1016/J.FORSCIINT.2009.03.034

[47] Can I, Javan GT, Pozhitkov AE, Noble PA. Distinctive thanatomicrobiome signatures found in the blood and internal organs of humans. Journal of Microbiological Methods. 2014;**106**:1-7. DOI: 10.1016/J.MIMET.2014.07.026

[48] Hyde ER, Haarmann DP, Lynne AM, Bucheli SR, Petrosino JF. The living dead: Bacterial community structure of a cadaver at the onset and end of the bloat stage of decomposition. PLoS One. 2013;**8**:e77733. DOI: 10.1371/journal.pone.0077733

[49] Tuomisto S, Pessi T, Collin P, Vuento R, Aittoniemi J, Karhunen PJ. Changes in gut bacterial populations and their translocation into liver and ascites in alcoholic liver cirrhotics. BMC Gastroenterology. 2014;**14**:40. DOI: 10.1186/1471-230X-14-40

[50] Javan GT, Finley SJ, Smith T, Miller J, Wilkinson JE. Cadaver thanatomicrobiome signatures: The ubiquitous nature of clostridium species in human decomposition. Frontiers in Microbiology. 2017;**8**:2096. DOI: 10.3389/fmicb.2017.02096

[51] Hu L, Xing Y, Jiang P, Gan L, Zhao F, Peng W, et al. Predicting the postmortem interval using human intestinal microbiome data and random forest algorithm. Science and Justice. 2021;**61**:516-527. DOI: 10.1016/j.scijus.2021.06.006

[52] Wallace JR, Receveur JP, Hutchinson PH, Kaszubinski SF, Wallace HE, Benbow ME. Microbial community succession on submerged vertebrate carcasses in a tidal river habitat: Implications for aquatic forensic investigations. Journal of Forensic Sciences. 2021;**66**:2307-2318. DOI: 10.1111/1556-4029.14869

[53] Houtz JL, Receveur JP, Pechal JL, Benbow ME, Horton BM, Wallace JR. Characterization of the avian postmortem gut microbiome across space and time using 16S rRNA sequencing. Forensic Science International: Animals and Environments. 2022;**2**:100053. DOI: 10.1016/J.FSIAE.2022.100053

[54] Zhao X, Zhong Z, Hua Z. Estimation of the post-mortem interval by modelling the changes in oral bacterial diversity during decomposition. Journal of Applied Microbiology. 2022;**133**(6):3451-3464. DOI: 10.1111/jam.15771

[55] Carter DO, Yellowlees D, Tibbett M. Temperature affects microbial decomposition of cadavers (Rattus rattus) in contrasting soils. Applied Soil Ecology. 2008;**40**:129-137. DOI: 10.1016/J.APSOIL.2008.03.010

[56] Carter DO, Yellowlees D, Tibbett M. Moisture can be the dominant environmental parameter governing cadaver decomposition in soil. Forensic Science International. 2010;**200**:60-66. DOI: 10.1016/J.FORSCIINT.2010.03.031

[57] Iancu L, Junkins EN, Necula-Petrareanu G, Purcarea C. Characterizing forensically important insect and microbial community colonization patterns in buried remains. Scientific Reports. 2018;**8**(1):15513. DOI: 10.1038/s41598-018-33794-0

[58] Javan GT, Finley SJ, Tuomisto S, Hall A, Benbow ME, Mills DE. An interdisciplinary review of the thanatomicrobiome in human decomposition. Forensic Science, Medicine, and Pathology. 2019;**15**:75-83. DOI: 10.1007/s12024-018-0061-0

[59] Hill GT, Mitkowski NA, Aldrich-Wolfe L, Emele LR, Jurkonie DD, Ficke A, et al. Methods for assessing the composition and diversity of soil microbial communities. Applied Soil Ecology. 2000;**15**:25-36. DOI: 10.1016/S0929-1393(00)00069-X

[60] Leung MHY, Wilkins D, Lee PKH. Insights into the pan-microbiome: Skin microbial communities of Chinese individuals differ from other racial groups. Scientific Reports. 2015;**5**:11845. DOI: 10.1038/srep11845

[61] Liu R, Gu Y, Shen M, Li H, Zhang K, Wang Q, et al. Predicting postmortem interval based on microbial community sequences and machine learning algorithms. Environmental Microbiology. 2020;**22**:2273-2291. DOI: 10.1111/1462-2920.15000

[62] Speruda M, Piecuch A, Borzęcka J, Kadej M, Ogórek R. Microbial traces and their role in forensic science. Journal of Applied Microbiology. 2022;**132**:2547-2557. DOI: 10.1111/JAM.15426

[63] Huttenhower C, Gevers D, Knight R, Abubucker S, Badger JH, Chinwalla AT, et al. The human microbiome project HMP consortium structure function and diversity of the healthy human microbiome. Nature. 2012;**486**:207-214. DOI: 10.1038/NATURE11234

[64] Dewhirst FE, Chen T, Izard J, Paster BJ, Tanner ACR, Yu WH, et al. The human Oral microbiome. Journal of Bacteriology. 2010;**192**:5002. DOI: 10.1128/JB.00542-10

[65] Gevers W. Biochemical aspects of cell death. Forensic Science. 1975;**6**:25-29. DOI: 10.1016/0300-9432(75)90220-4

[66] Schmitt A, Cunha E, Pinheiro J. Forensic Anthropology and Medicine: Complementary Sciences from Recovery to Cause of Death. Totowa, New Jersey: Humana Press; 2006. DOI: 10.1007/978-1-59745-099-7

[67] Metcalf JL, Xu ZZ, Weiss S, Lax S, Van Treuren W, Hyde ER, et al.

Microbial community assembly and metabolic function during mammalian corpse decomposition. Science. 1979;**2016**(351):158-162. DOI: 10.1126/science.aad2646

[68] Procopio N, Ghignone S, Williams A, Chamberlain A, Mello A, Buckley M. Metabarcoding to investigate changes in soil microbial communities within forensic burial contexts. Forensic Science International. Genetics. 2019;**39**:73-85. DOI: 10.1016/J.FSIGEN.2018.12.002

Chapter 3

Limited Approaches for Genomic Studies in Rapid Postmortem Tissue Collection

George Sandusky, Michael Yard, Megan Szymanski, Lydia Emmert and Vivian Valadares

Abstract

Rapid postmortem tissue collection has been shown to have increasing use for molecular and genetic profiling. Although research on human tissue has been conducted for many years, modern molecular assays have significantly higher sensitivity and specificity than those used in the past. Higher grade tissue specimens are now required for the extraction of macromolecules as a result of this. In fact, these studies have paved the way for multiple postmortem tissue collection studies such as COVID-19, brain, skin, and small cell lung cancer. Best practices for tissue collection have also been developed by a number of professional organizations, including the National Institutes of Health Office of Biorepositories and the International Society of Biological and Environmental Repositories (ISBER). These guidelines can be used to establish procedures for tissue collection.

Keywords: autopsy, post-mortem, COVID-19, small cell lung cancer, SCLC, skin, histology, post-mortem interval, RIN

1. Introduction

One of the most important tools for the study of human disease and the creation of new therapeutics is human tissue specimens. The techniques utilized for sample collecting and processing can have a significant impact on the molecular information included in tissue samples. Several factors that are essential for collecting high-quality tissues are covered in this chapter. By adhering to pre-established guidelines and standard operating procedures, tissue samples will be handled consistently and optimally, minimizing the impact of environmental factors on a sample's quality and molecular profile.

2. Tissue collection for genomic research

2.1 Tissue collection

Proper collection and preservation of tissue specimens is fundamental to the ability to isolate enough high-quality nucleic acids for genomic research. It is now well-recognized that changes in the molecular profile of a tissue can occur during sample retrieval, between the time interval from retrieval to processing, and during processing itself. Therefore, it is important to establish standardized guidelines that keep the time from specimen collection to preservation as short as possible and maintain consistency in the handling of samples.

One of the major factors influencing the integrity of nucleic acids in stored tissue samples is tissue ischemia time. The surgical disruption of blood flow to an excised clinical sample leads to progressive tissue ischemia, hypoxia, and release of endogenous nuclease enzymes capable of degrading nucleic acids. The warm ischemia time is the time from the interruption of the blood supply to the removal of a tissue sample from the patient, while the cold ischemia time is the time from removal of a tissue to its preservation by freezing or by placement in a fixative. Warm ischemia time is dependent on the surgery and can be difficult to control. In contrast, the institution's tissue collection and transportation protocols affect the cold ischemia time and can be readily controlled using standardized sample collection and handling procedures. To minimize tissue and cell damage, the cold ischemia time should be kept as short as possible. It is important that both the warm and cold ischemia times are documented [1, 2].

2.2 Tissue preservation and storage

In general, three basic methods of sample preservation exist: snap freezing, fixation, and a nucleic acid stabilizing reagent. If enough material is available, it is often advisable to split and preserve the tissue sample using multiple methods (e.g. snap freeze half the tissue and fix the other half in formalin).

Fresh-frozen tissue samples provide optimal quality nucleic acids, compared to fixed tissue specimens. However, the freezing process can compromise tissue morphology, so this method is not always ideal if tissue morphology is to be examined. The process of snap-freezing may also pose logistical issues for some laboratories because it requires specialized equipment. Snap-freezing (also known as flash freezing) is the process by which samples are lowered to temperatures below −70°C very rapidly. Snap-freezing, as opposed to standard freezing, reduces the chances of water in the sample forming ice crystals and damaging the tissue. Snap-freezing also slows the actions of nucleases and proteases thus inhibiting the degradation of nucleic acids and protein in the sample.

If examination of tissue morphology by histochemical or immunohistochemical means is required, formalin fixation and paraffin embedding (FFPE) is the standard process for sample preservation. The FFPE process not only preserves tissue morphology, but also allows for easy transport and storage and permanent preservation of the tissue. Formalin fixation is carried out by submerging the tissue specimen directly in 10% neutral-buffered formalin (NBF) at room temperature. For molecular assays, the optimal fixation time is approximately 14–18 h. Studies have shown that longer fixation times tend to result in poor quality RNA.

Another common method of preservation is submersion of the tissue directly in a nucleic acid stabilizing reagent such as PAXgene® Tissue Fix, TRIzol or RNAlater. This method is ideal for minimizing nucleic acid damage and changes in gene expression.

2.3 Use of wet ice for stabilization of genomic RNA

One method of transporting organs is through the use of wet ice. One pilot cardiovascular study collecting explanted hearts from 1996 to 2008 experimented using this method. There were 50 heart explants from the heart transplant team. The explanted hearts were delivered to the surgical pathology gross room by the heart team. The heart was then packed in a stainless-steel surgical bucket of wet crushed ice using the three-bag technique. The heart was washed in transplant solution before putting the first bag in preservation solution which was patented by University of Wisconsin. The heart was dissected with approximately half the sections being transferred into 10% NBF and the other half into small containers surrounded by wet ice for transportation to the processing lab. The tissue samples were placed in an −80° C freezer and put into a liquid nitrogen tank. Research at the time did not fully support the use of wet ice for preservation of RNA; however, this study found that the RIN quality was not impacted by using wet ice. Other studies worked with four different organ procurement organizations (OPO) in Indianapolis for about 10 years and found the same preservation of RNA in wet ice yielded high RIN values [3–7].

2.4 Histology quality control

Quality control analysis begins at the histology level and should be performed real-time as tissue specimens are received. For each procured tissue, a hematoxylin and eosin (H&E)-stained slide should be generated and reviewed under a microscope. In the case of tumor specimens, the pathologist confirms that the sample contains enough tumor cells (at least 50%) to be considered acceptable for molecular analysis. Tumor samples that contain less than 50% tumor might be released only for applications, such as immunohistochemistry or in situ hybridization. In addition to evaluating the percentage of viable tumor cells, guidelines issued by ISBER and NCI state the pathologist should also make note of the percentages of necrosis, fibrosis, mucin formation, stroma, normal adjacent tissue, and inflammation [8–13].

2.5 Nucleic acid quality control

Archival FFPE samples are notorious for yielding poor-quality nucleic acids after 5 years of storage. Therefore, it is important to evaluate the molecular quality of each sample before its release for subsequent molecular testing. For retention of high-quality RNA, freezing is currently the best method of long-term tissue storage. Although not as labile as RNA, DNA molecules are also susceptible to degradation during the long-term storage of tissue samples [8–10].

2.6 Post-mortem specimens

Post-mortem human tissues are a valuable source of biological material. These specimens have versatile research applications, but the quality must be maintained throughout processing. In animal studies, the handling and storage of tissues immediately after death can be easily controlled. However, in human studies, the uncontrollability of these factors leads to a higher degree of variability. For example, the time lag between death and preservation of a sample following autopsy (PMI) is a major factor influencing the quality of RNA in post-mortem tissues. Existing evidence suggests that there is little correlation between the post-mortem interval and RNA quality/ RIN score. The integrity of RNA in post-mortem samples appears to be linked to pre-mortem factors such as the cause of death and the length and duration of the period just before death, known as the agonal period.

3. Background of pilot RNA post-mortem study

3.1 Introduction

Numerous research studies have analyzed the post-mortem brain tissue's quality. When analyzing post-mortem brain tissue, the goal of genetic research has been to comprehend neurological illnesses. These investigations have made significant progress and identified high RNA quality [14, 15]. These studies recorded pre-mortem fever or sepsis, pre-mortem tissue pH, temporal relationship to time of death (either sudden death or protracted illness), post-mortem interval, and other significant health conditions prior to death [16]. In the last 10 years, the integrity and general quality of the tissue have been assessed using the quality of the RNA. RNA quality is currently assessed using electrophoresis and RIN values [17]. The length of time before death till tissue removal, the classification of death, and the state of the patient's health before death all may have an impact on the quality of the RNA in the tissue [18].

In addition to RNA quality assessed by RIN values, the area of postmortem neuropathology has developed chemical markers for tissue quality, starting with pH and the 28S/18S ratio. Ten organ tissues from four postmortem instances with various PMI were examined. To ascertain the histology and molecular markers of the postmortem tissue, the clinical history, agonal condition, refrigeration time, and PMI of 10, 12, 16, and >24 h were assessed (**Figure 1**) [18].

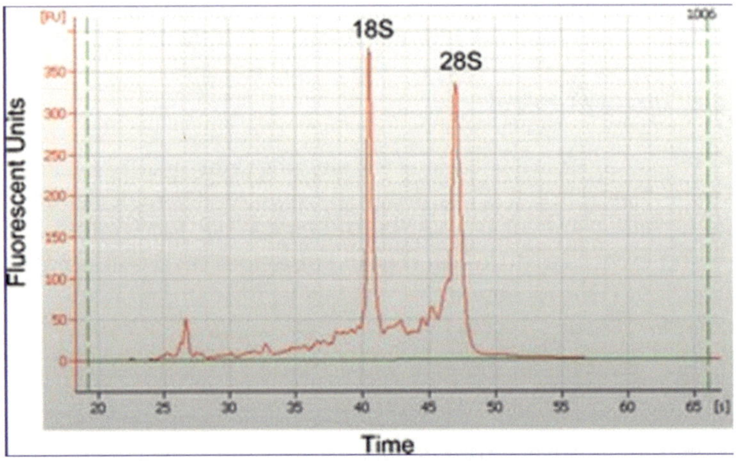

Figure 1.
Tissue RNA evaluation using a whole electrophoretogram to quantitate a RIN value.

3.2 Results

RNA stability (RIN values) was not predicted by the PMI, although cooling after death affected body temperature, postponed post-mortem autolysis, and improved RIN levels. However, RIN values fell with sustained hypoxemia. Two of the key factors influencing RIN values were agonal state scores and clinical medical history. RIN values decreased when agonal state scores were high, which is consistent with previous research. Most organs' RIN scores could be predicted from histology, with the exception of the pancreas and small intestine, which autolyzed relatively quickly. RIN values for all organs are shown in **Table 1**.

This study was used as a pilot for the following ongoing human genomic studies: suicidality [19], small cell lung cancer, COVID-19 [20], and skin [21]. As a result of the pilot study for the GTEx tissue collection study, multiple

Tissue	A	B	C	D	Average
Liver	3	4.9	2.5	7.7	4.5
Kidney	7.2	2.9	3.4	4.1	4.4
Heart	8.2	6.8	7.7	5.8	7.1
Lung	5.6	5.8	5.1	7	5.9
Small Intestine	5.2	6.4	3.6	5.5	5.2
Pancreas	4.7	2.6	1.8	2.7	3
Skin	7.4	3.6	4.6	7.8	5.9
Brain	7.9	4.5	4.7	N/C	N/C
Cerebellum	8.7	3.9	N/C	5.3	N/C
Skeletal muscle	8.3	N/C	N/C	N/C	N/C
Bone marrow	2.7	2.9	N/C	3	N/C

Table 1.
Breakdown of patients A-D RIN values [18].

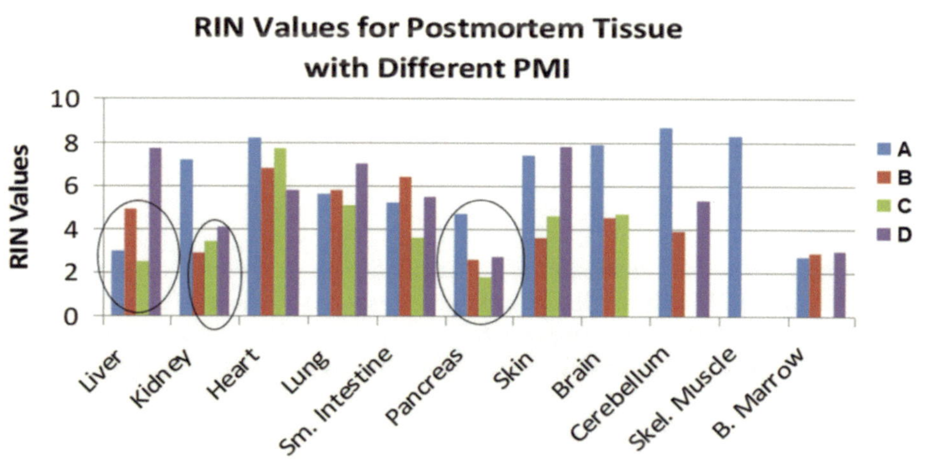

Figure 2.
Patients A-D RIN values for each tissue collected [18].

Patient	A	B	C	D
Refrigeration (h)	4.80	2.10	9.80	0.13
Refrigeration Time (h)	23.55	14.50	2.17	9.17
Refrigeration to Autopsy (h)	0.33	0.25	0.23	0.25
Total time (h)	28.68	16.85	12.20	9.55

Table 2.
Comparison of patients A-D PMI intervals [18].

Patient	Agonal score	Agonal factors
A	3	Failed bone marrow transplant for multiple myeloma
B	1	CO_2 Poisoning
C	2	Wound (more detail later)
D	3	48 h medically-induced hypothermia during brain death protocol

Table 3.
Agonal state score and factors of patients A-D [18].

studies involving genomic expression in esophageal carcinoma, lung adenocarcinoma, and breast tumors have been conducted (**Figure 2** and **Tables 2** and **3**) [1, 2, 3, 18, 21].

4. Methodological considerations of brain and blood recovery, analysis, and storage

4.1 Introduction

The proper methodology for recovery, analyzing, and storage of human specimens is a common source of discussion among many scientists and researchers across the world. Many intrinsic and extrinsic factors such as temperature, timeliness of collection, and natural disease processes influence the quality of tissue, and thus the effectiveness to which the specimen can be analyzed. This section will discuss our SOP for brain banking and biological fluid in this brain collection. In general, our process includes protocols for the recovery, analysis, and storage of sections and entire brain specimens.

4.2 Methods used

Three main methods of collection in the suicidality project were used: blood collection, DNA, and RNA tubes. All methods were designed to allow an easy medium to which DNA and/or RNA may be extracted and analyzed. Blood was generally collected in PAXgene® DNA and RNA tubes due to their long ambient temperature requirements.

The SOP began with deputy coroners/hospital staff notifying staff of a death that fits collection criteria guidelines. A taped verbal consent was obtained from the next of kin by action of the Deputy coroner and Followed up with obtaining signed written informed consent at the morgue or at the funeral home by the Coroner's

Office. Once these two actions were completed, the case was approved for tissue and/or blood collection.

The reagents include 4 mL labeled and bar-coded tubes for storage via PAX Gene tubes for RNA and DNA. If possible, whole blood was collected from normal patients and patients with neurological diseases. Tissue procurement included collection of PAXgene® DNA and RNA tubes from the subclavian vein or heart, removal of calvarium, documentation and photography of whole brain weight, cutting and sectioning of brain, and prompt freezing of samples at −80° C.

Prolonged ischemic state of brain tissue, natural disease processes such as Alzheimer's disease, and long postmortem intervals may have affected the quality of recovery of brain tissue and RIN values. While pH premortem acidosis often influenced viable brain tissue for genomic studies, pH is stable post-mortem and during consequent freezer storage. Typically, individuals who suffered prolonged agonal states tended to have more acidotic brains. Conversely, those who experienced brief deaths typically had a normal pH. RIN values in most postmortem tissues is highly correlated with medical history and agonal state. Natural disease processes and length of time taken to collect specimens after the decedent's passing are taken into consideration. Special consideration was taken for subjects with a history of psychiatric disorders, psychiatric visits and hospitalizations, suicide attempts, and excessive use of alcohol and/or street drugs.

The inclusion and exclusion criteria were then further examined. Inclusion criteria consisted of the decedent's medical history being consistent with schizophrenia, schizoaffective disorder, bipolar disorder, major depression, a postmortem interval of 24 h or less, any gender or race, 18 years or older (unless otherwise agreed upon in writing by a legal representative of the decedent), and appropriate informed consent forms. Oppositely, the exclusion criteria included greater than a 24 h post mortem interval, any primary or metastatic brain cancer, history of stroke, intracranial bleed or other brain trauma, severe alcoholism or Korsakoff's syndrome, history of congenital brain defects, sepsis, infection, communicable disease, prolonged hypoxia or intubation/ventilator assisted breathing for greater than 12 hs, use of vasopressors prior to death, and attempted ACLS resuscitation.

Staff also developed strict quality control criteria. Upon each new sample obtained, the following quality control checks are performed: RIN ≥ 7.0 for frozen specimens, pH ≥ 6, proper FFPE specimen fixation, and appropriate preparation, labeling, and storage of samples, specimens, and data [19].

4.3 Concern for biohazard material

All human specimens should be considered potential biohazards whether they are fixed, paraffin-embedded, or fresh frozen. Due to the hazardous nature of the organs under examination, universal precaution was taken and standard procedures were implemented while handling the specimens.

4.4 Collection of brain

In addition to removal of the brain, factors of concern included the weight of the whole brain, bleeding, prior healed or open/partly open surgical incisions of the scalp or skull bone, dura stuck inside the calvarium or if it peeled away from the skull and stuck on the brain, and whether the surface of the meninges were stained with blood or were transparent. If any of these conditions were observed, the location and severeness of the afflictions were noted and photographed for documentation purposes.

The entire brain, including the cerebrum, cerebellum, and brain stem, are removed per standard autopsy procedure (**Figures 3** and **4**). The brain was then placed in a plastic bag partially filled with saline and placed in an ice-filled cooler. Upon arrival at the designated grossing area, the brain was divided by a mid-sagittal cut through the corpus callosum. A coronal sectioning was also performed through the brain hemisphere from anterior to posterior.

Next, a section of the identified region is cut that is approximately 1 cm thick. The section is then trisected to create three samples that are approximately 3 mm thick. Samples in the cassettes are then transported on wet ice and immediately (within 15 min) placed in a – 80°C freezer. The time that each sample is frozen is recorded. The last remaining sample is then placed into a white cassette and immediately placed in 10% neutral buffered formalin.

4.5 Storage of brain tissue

A pH strip was placed on the first section (about 10 seconds) to get the pH of the brain. Subsequent slices were made parallel to the first cut, producing 14 slices. The slices were then placed on a blue cutting board and photographed with a digital camera. Slices were slowly frozen using cooled stainless-steel plates. The precooled plates were then placed on ice packs in a flat Styrofoam container. Slight pressure on the upper stainless-steel plate allowed the cut brain slices to flatten out. More ice packs were then placed on top of the upper stainless-steel plate.

4.6 Conclusion

The data pertaining to all cases were compiled in a single database spreadsheet. Also present at each site for procurement, analysis, and storage are data books used to update the research study with pertinent findings and basic demographics. There

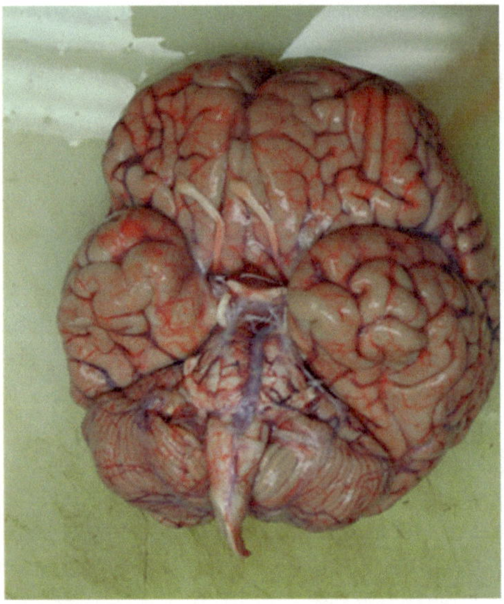

Figure 3.
Whole brain removed after prosection.

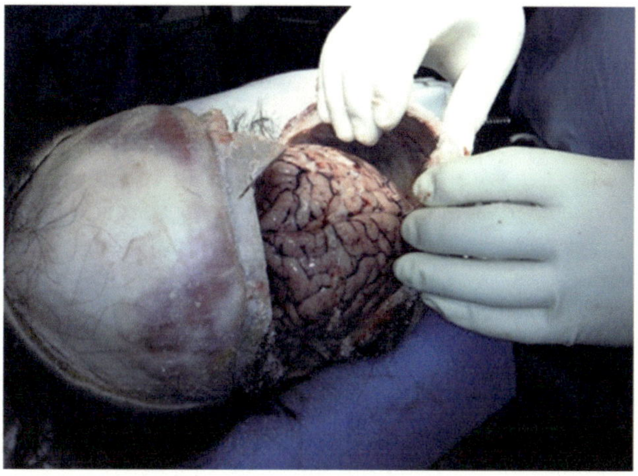

Figure 4.
Incision from ear to ear of decedent is then reflected in order to remove calvarium. Temporalis muscles removed in order for autopsy bone saw to properly cut through calvarium.

were 180 total cases collected under the suicidality protocol and we had high-quality RNA data from blood samples. After seven brains were collected, we compared RNA profile from both brain and blood. Past findings showed the mutated genes were similar. The brain collection was stopped after the seventh case and are now only collecting DNA and RNA blood samples in PAXgene® tubes.

5. Collection of lung and blood for COVID-19 post-mortem study

5.1 Introduction

In the past 3 years, a novel acute respiratory RNA virus known as SARS-Cov-2 has grown into a pandemic. In this investigation, the lung pathology of 43 individuals who passed away and displayed significant COVID-19 symptoms was examined. Decedents were not seen in a clinical environment and were taken post-mortem. Decedents ranged in age from 3 to 76 years old. Ethnicities included 29 Caucasians, eight African American, three Hispanic, one Cuban, one Asian, and one unknown. There was a male to female ratio of 4:1. All cases were classified into positive and negative COVID-19 using the FDA and CDC approved RT-PCR test. Eighteen were negative and twenty-one were positive for COVID. A subset of these cases (11) was positive for cocaine, methamphetamine, fentanyl, morphine, acetyl fentanyl, chronic ethanol, or sertraline. There were additional compounding etiologies with most of these cases (diabetes, trauma, and atherosclerotic heart disease) [22].

5.2 Concern for biohazard material

All human specimens should be considered as potential biohazards whether they are fixed, paraffin-embedded, or fresh frozen. Due to the hazardous nature of the organs under examination, universal precaution standard procedures were implemented while handling the specimens.

5.3 Tissue specimens

Informed consent and IRB approval was obtained. All lung and blood samples were collected at the Marion County Coroner's Office. These were partial intercostal surgeries with a biological fluid blood draw over the period of April 9, 2020 to March 15, 2021.

Body transport: The body was transported from the scene of death to Marion County Morgue. The group used Tyvek Iso Clean surgical gowns over scrub suits, thick rubber gloves, surgical masks, eye goggle protection, surgical boots, and surgical slippers.

Lung removal: The clavicle was identified (rib 1 beneath clavicle) and counted down to ribs 3–5. An incision was made through the skin and through the thoracic cage from the mid-axillary line over to the manubrium of the sternum between ribs 4–7. This incision was approximately 10–12 cm in length. A vacuum was used to remove any fluid from the chest cavity. A small piece of lung tissue from the right middle lobe (5 cm × 7 cm) was removed and placed in 10% NBF. PAXgene® DNA and RNA blood samples were drawn from the superior vena cava.

For this infectious disease lung study, lung tissues were fixed at 4°C for 48 h, instead of the usual 18 h followed by tissue processing, embedding in paraffin, and staining for H&E and Trichrome. Approximately 14 sections of lung were collected from each case.

Immunology: Antibodies were tested in various cases. Total RNA isolation was performed on all samples.

RNA extraction: RNA QC and qRT-PCR were used to confirm viral load in all 23 positive deceased blood and lung samples. The average post-mortem interval for these samples was 14 ½ h.

5.4 Findings

The findings were similar to previous COVID-19 findings. We had both acute and chronic inflammation in the lung samples. The histology in the acute cases were characterized by minimal bronchiolar perivascular lymphocytic infiltration, focal hyaline membrane formation, severe pulmonary congestion, bronchiolar respiratory epithelial/alveolar pneumocyte necrosis, formation of microthrombi, and pulmonary edema. Interstitial pneumonia with thickening of the alveolar wall, perivascular and peribronchiolar lymphocytic infiltration, multifocal areas of fibroplasia, microthrombi, severe congestion, squamous metaplasia of the alveolar epithelium, and fibrosis and septal collagen deposition were the hallmarks of the histology in the chronic cases.

We performed immunohistochemistry using both DNA and fluorescence imaging of lung tissue and detection of the COVID-19 virus. In addition, total RNA isolation with qRT-PCR and RNA Seq was completed to confirm the diseased blood in lung samples.

6. Collection of liver and lung for small cell lung cancer study

6.1 Introduction

This study examined a rapid autopsy program including three patients currently looking for mutational and molecular changes in small cell lung cancer (SCLC). The findings will provide new insights into treatment resistance and lead to new targets to find more effective immunotherapy and targeted therapies for advanced SCLC. SCLC is one of the rarest types of lung cancer, affecting 10–15% of all patients with lung cancer. Diagnosis usually occurs once the patient is symptomatic and after metastasis has occurred. It has one of the worst prognoses out of all lung cancers and is the hardest to treat. Blood samples from the superior vena cava were collected in the funeral home in order to keep the PMI under 8 h. Two more cases are currently being processed using this protocol. Most autopsy rooms do not collect tissue after usual business hours, and we have done all collections in a funeral home.

6.2 Specimen collection

Blood collection was performed utilizing the subclavian vein. Six tubes were collected: DNA, RNA, Peripheral blood mononuclear cells (PBMCs), Natural Killer (NK), circulating tumor cells (CTC), and In Vivo were collected (**Figure 4**). PAXgene® DNA and RNA were collected for stability purposes.

MRIs were performed to determine an appropriate location for lung and liver collection. Lung removal was characterized by an incision of 10–12 cm made through the skin through the mid-axillary line over to the manubrium of the sternum between ribs 3–7. Rib retractors were used to spread the ribs and have a large field to visualize the lesions in the lungs (**Figure 5**). Russian tissue forceps were used to remove the mass and adjacent normal tissue. A scalpel and/or autopsy knife is then used to dissect mass into 250–750 mg sample sizes. Masses were transferred to 10% neutral buffered formalin (NBF) and MACS solution.

Liver removal was characterized by an incision of 10–12 cm made below the xiphoid process. The skin and fascia were lifted utilizing Russian tissue forceps, and a scalpel was used to cut into fascia. Liver palpation was performed to identify the mass and was carefully cut along with normal adjacent tissue. A vacuum to remove excess fluid accumulation from the abdominal cavity was used if necessary. Samples sizes of 250–750 mg were transferred into 10% NBF and transported on wet ice.

6.3 Subclavian vein location

The following anatomical landmarks were identified. The sternocleidomastoid muscle insertion into the clavicle was visible. Below the clavicle is the right subclavian

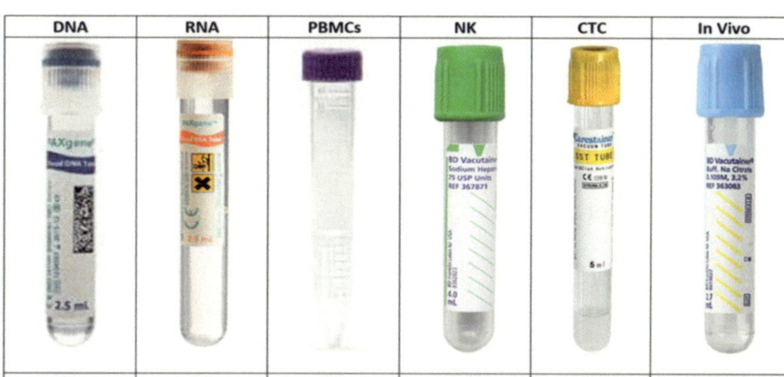

Figure 5.
Visual illustration of order of collection of blood tubes.

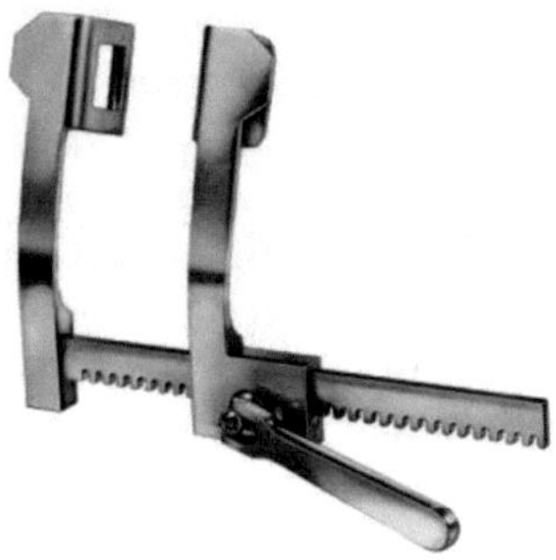

Figure 6.
Rib spreader.

vein. At the top of the ribcage, the right subclavian vein starts. The skin puncture site can be identified by landmarks 1 cm laterally from the sternocleidomastoid muscle's posterior clavicular head and 1 cm down under from the clavicle (**Figure 6**).

7. Collection of skin specimen

7.1 Introduction

The Post-mortem Tissue Collection Skin Project has collected 80 cases to date. Tissue collection was completed by the Marion County Coroner's Office, and from there was transported on wet ice to the regenerative medicine lab where the skin samples were fixed and embedded into paraffin blocks. Skin samples were collected and divided into two samples. One went into 10% NBF and the other into MACS solution. MACS solution was kept in wet ice as it was transferred to the research lab. Microscope slides were prepared and stained with hematoxylin and eosin (H&E) and Masson's Trichrome for autolysis detection. In addition, Visium spatial gene expression slides were created for molecular profiling. Tissues were profiled on a 4-point Hardy Score (**Figures 7** and **8**).

7.2 Specimen collection

Skin specimens are identified with an alpha-numeric Specimen ID that contains the case ID and a sequence number. Collection time should stay under 16 h. A sun-exposed (e.g., lower limbs) 6x3 cm strip of skin is collected and cut into two sections. The tissue is preserved in MACS solution and PAXgene® tissue fixative and transferred over wet ice to the lab. After collection, the Sample Collection Form is filled out and the drug data is collected from the deputy coroner, such as cause of death, toxicology, and prescription pills report.

7.3 Results

MACS solution separated the dermal collagen fibers in the dermis compared to the PAXgene® tissue fix. Initially, a PMI of 8 h was used, but after analysis of six samples it was expanded to 12 h and then to 16 h. At 16 h, the genetic material was superior quality with high RIN values (>6).

[1] Death classification based on the 4-point Hardy Scale:
0: Ventilator Case All cases on a ventilator immediately before death.
1: Violent and fast death due to accident, blunt force trauma or suicide, terminal phase estimated at < 10 min.
2: Fast death of natural causes. Sudden unexpected deaths of people who had been reasonably healthy, after a terminal phase estimated at < 1 hr (with sudden death from a myocardial infarction as a model cause of death for this category).
3: Intermediate death. Death after a terminal phase of 1 to 24 hrs (not classifiable as 2 or 4); patients who were ill but death was unexpected.
4: Slow death. Death after a long illness, with a terminal phase longer than 1 day (commonly cancer or chronic pulmonary disease); deaths that are not unexpected.
[2] The destruction of organism cells or tissues by the organisms' own enzymes or processes.
[3] See Schroeder A, Mueller O, Stocker S, et al. The RIN: an RNA integrity number for assigning integrity values to RNA measurements. *BMC molecular biology*. Jan 31 2006;7:3

Figure 7.
Description of 4-point hardy scale.

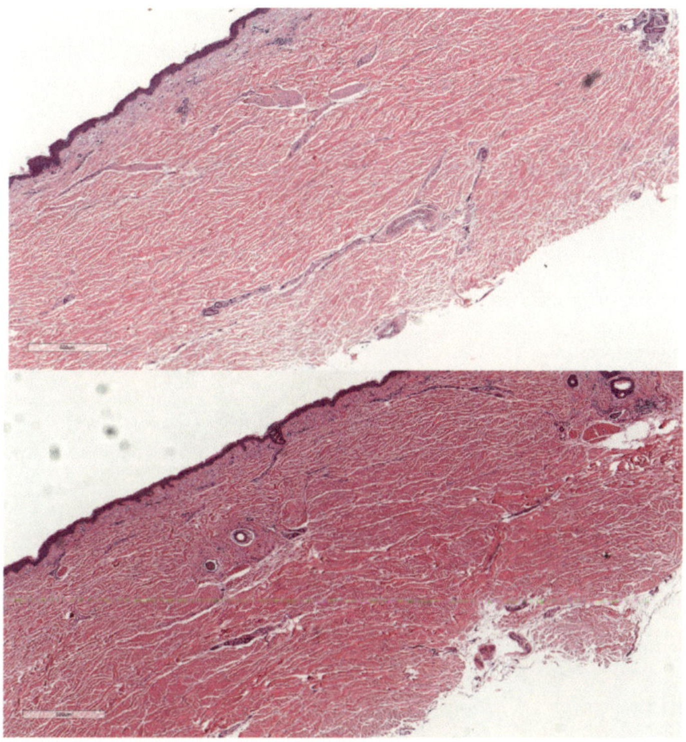

Figure 8.
Skin collected in MACS solution (top) compared to PAXgene® tissue fix (bottom).

8. Conclusions

In recent years, the development of new molecular technologies with improved specificity, sensitivity, and throughput has greatly increased the demand for high quality, well-annotated biological specimens. By using surgical techniques instead of traditional autopsy protocols, we were able to maintain a short PMI and high genomic quality for samples collected. We have been able to collect tissues such as skin, lungs, and blood, advancing the research of post-mortem human genomics.

Acknowledgements

Thanks to Mikayla Stephens, Sarah Seibert, Kayli Nguyen, Maggie Granatir, Jessica Jackson, Matt Rodgers, Frank Lloyd, Dean Hawley, Rebekah Addison, Madelynn Gaines, Kanhaiya Singh, Chandan Sen, Charles Saller, and Raymond Howanski. We appreciate everyone who took the time to contribute to this research and the Marion County Coroner's Office.

Conflict of interest

The authors declare no conflict of interest.

Author details

George Sandusky*, Michael Yard, Megan Szymanski, Lydia Emmert and Vivian Valadares
IU School of Medicine, Indiana University-Purdue University Indianapolis, Indianapolis, IN, USA

*Address all correspondence to: gsandusk@iupui.edu

References

[1] Cancer Genome Atlas Research Network...Sandusky GE. Integrated genomic characterization of oesophageal carcinoma. Nature. 2017;**541**(7636):169-175. DOI: 10.1038/nature20805

[2] Cancer Genome Atlas Research Network...Sandusky GE. Comprehensive molecular profiling of lung adenocarcinoma. Nature. 2014;**511**(7511):543-550. DOI: 10.1038/nature13385

[3] Sandusky GE, Offen JC, Clark MA. A survey of human myocarditis cases diagnosed using Alexa immunofluorescence dyes and confocal microscopy. Life Science Journal. 2006;**3**(4):37-41

[4] Spencer C, Carr KA, Mitchell C, Sandusky GE. Quality control from a subset of human surgical tissue specimens from the IU Simon Cancer Center Tissue Bank collected in 2009-2010. In: An H&E and RIN Value Assessment: ISBER Annual Mtg; May 2011; Washington, DC. 2011

[5] Sandusky GE, Clark MA. Heart Transplantation and Evaluation of the Heart Explant. Madison, Wisconsin: University of Wisconsin; 2007

[6] Sandusky GE, Clark MA. Hypertrophic Cardiomyopathy: Midwest Pathology. Columbus, Ohio: Ohio State University; 2008

[7] Sandusky GE, Clark MA. Idiopathic Cardiomyopathy: Midwest Pathology. West Lafayette, IN: Purdue University; 2009

[8] Stan AD, Ghose S, Gao X, Roberts RC, Lewis-Amezcua K, Hatanpaa KJ, et al. Human post-mortem tissue: What quality markers matter? Brain Research. 2006;**1123**(1):1-11. DOI: 10.1016/j.brainres.2006.09.025

[9] Preece P, Cairns NJ. Quantifying mRNA in post-mortem human brain: Influence of gender, age at death, post-mortem interval, brain pH, agonal state and inter-lobe mRNA variance. Brain Research. Molecular Brain Research. 2003;**118**(1-2):60-71. DOI: 10.1016/s0169-328x(03)00337-1

[10] Hynd MR, Lewohl JM, Scott HL, Dodd PR. Biochemical and molecular studies using human autopsy brain tissue. Journal of Neurochemistry. 2003;**85**(3):543-562. DOI: 10.1046/j.1471-4159.2003.01747.x

[11] International Society for Biological and Environmental Repositories. Best Practices: Recommendations for Repositories. 4th ed. Biopreserv Biobank; 2018

[12] National Cancer Institute. Best Practices for Biospecimen Resources. U.S. Department of Health and Human Services, National Institutes of Health. 2016

[13] Sandusky GE, Teheny KH, Esterman M, Hanson J, Williams SD. Quality control of human tissues--experience from the Indiana University Cancer Center-Lilly Research Labs human tissue bank. Cell and Tissue Banking. 2007;**8**(4):287-295. Epub 2007 Mar 27

[14] Catts VS, Catts SV, Fernandez HR, Taylor JM, Coulson EJ, Lutze-Mann LH. A microarray study of post-mortem mRNA degradation in mouse brain tissue. Brain Research. Molecular Brain Research. 2005;**138**(2):164-177. DOI: 10.1016/j.molbrainres.2005.04.017

[15] Cummings TJ, Strum JC, Yoon LW, Szymanski MH, Hulette CM. Recovery and expression of messenger RNA from post-mortem human brain tissue. Modern Pathology. 2001;**14**(11):1157-1161. DOI: 10.1038/modpathol.3880451

[16] Lipska BK, Deep-Soboslay A, Weickert CS, Hyde TM, Martin CE, Herman MM, et al. Critical factors in gene expression in post-mortem human brain: Focus on studies in schizophrenia. Biological Psychiatry. 2006;**60**(6):650-658. DOI: 10.1016/j.biopsych.2006.06.019

[17] Lee J, Hever A, Willhite D, Zlotnik A, Hevezi P. Effects of RNA degradation on gene expression analysis of human post-mortem tissues. The FASEB Journal. 2005;**19**(10):1356-1358. DOI: 10.1096/fj.04-3552fje

[18] Szymanski M, Hawley D, Sandusky GE. Investigating the correlation between post-mortem interval and RIN values: A pilot study. International Journal of Nursing Research. 2023;**6**:1444. DOI: 10.29011/2688-9501.101444

[19] Le-Niculescu H, Levey DF, Ayalew M, Palmer L, Gavrin LM, Jain N, et al. Discovery and validation of blood biomarkers for suicidality. Molecular Psychiatry. 2013;**18**(12):1249-1264. DOI: 10.1038/mp.2013.95

[20] Abouhashem AS, Singh K, Srivastava R, Liu S, Steiner S, Gu X, et al. The prolonged terminal phase of human life induces survival response in the skin transcriptome. BioRxiv. 2023. DOI: 10.1101%2F2023.05.15.540715

[21] The GTEx Consortium. The genotype-tissue expression (GTEx) project. Nature Genetics. 2013;**45**(6):580-585. DOI: 10.1038/ng.2653

[22] Bloom A, Colter A, Jacobsen M, Battles D, Albertson T, Sandusky G. Pathological lung lesions of COVID-19 and opioid use disorder: A post-mortem lung and toxicology examination of 43 decedents. FMAR. 2022;**10**(04):65-76. DOI: 10.4236/fmar.2022.104007

Chapter 4

Recovery and Rehydration of Decomposed and Mummified Tissues in Postmortem Analysis

William Aguilar-Navarro and Carmen Cerda-Aguilar

Abstract

After the death of individuals, sequential degradative processes called autolysis and putrefaction are initiated in the tissues, processes that cause total or partial degradation, sometimes leaving remnants of tissue. Mummification is a process by which the degradative processes are slowed and, in some cases, stopped, allowing the tissue to be apparently preserved. There are two main types of mummification: natural and artificial; natural mummification is caused by conditions related to the environment in which the tissues are located. Within the artificial techniques, there is cadaveric preservation (embalming), a procedure currently used for health and scientific studies. To carry out studies of tissues in some degree of decomposition or mummified, it is necessary to submit the samples for a process called recovery and/or rehydration, by means of immersion techniques in hypotonic solutions, which facilitates the processing and subsequent analysis of the characteristics of these tissues, both macroscopically and microscopically.

Keywords: decomposition, mummification, recovery, rehydration, analysis

1. Introduction

Tissues present a characteristic process of decomposition after the death of the individual; these processes are responsible for degrading the tissue in most cases until its complete disappearance [1]. However, depending on the multiple factors and conditions to which they are subjected, there are tissues in which the decomposition is altered; due to these changes, the tissues can be analyzed by subjecting them to some kind of recovery process.

The tissue preservation phenomena, one of which is the mummification process, corresponds to the dehydration of tissues, in which the whole body, segments, or tissues are apparently maintained in a certain state of preservation characterized by dehydration, hardening and a stiffened appearance of the tissues, a state that gives the impression that they have been preserved. This process delays or may halt the characteristic processes occurring during decomposition. Mummification can occur in two ways: spontaneous or natural and anthropogenic or artificial. The natural mummification process is influenced by factors such as environmental conditions, such as climate, air currents, chemical characteristics of the soil, factors that favor natural mummification [2]. In the process of artificial mummification, there are a series of procedures carried out on the corpse such as the addition of chemical fixatives in order to preserve the body in a certain state for as long as possible.

For postmortem analysis of tissues in initial state of decomposition or mummified, from a macroscopic or microscopic point of view, it is necessary to take the tissues and subject them to processes that allow them to return their structural integrity. Obtaining, as far as possible, results like those of a normal tissue, since the limiting factor of adequate results corresponds to the initial conditions in which the sample to be recovered is found. Conditions such as stage of tissue degradation, degree of mummification, more desiccated tissues are more difficult to recover, among many other factors.

2. Postmortem changes in tissues

When working with decomposing or mummified tissues, it is necessary to know the postmortem phenomena and how these are affected by various factors, such as body size and condition, tissue type, environmental temperature, soil porosity, chemical reactivity, pH, micro-organisms, and so on [1]. In the initial phase of postmortem phenomena, there are chemical changes in which enzymes play an important role, which due to their lytic activity produce the breakdown of macromolecules such as proteins, carbohydrates, and fatty acids, a phenomenon known as autolysis [3].

The breakdown of soft tissues is separated into three consecutive stages of enzymatic action, the first by tissue enzymes, the second by bacterial enzymes, and the third by insect action [2]. The tissue enzymes involved are hydrolytic and determine the self-digestion of the tissue [4]. The second stage in tissue degeneration is known as "putrefaction," given by endogenous or exogenous bacterial enzymatic activity, establishing the process of liquefaction and gasification of the tissues involved [5].

The emanation of various types of gases allows the arrival of other organisms such as insects and scavengers, which contribute to the decomposition process by definitively degrading the tissues [6]. As tissue decomposition requires certain conditions specific to the cellular and tissue environment, such as availability of water, humidity, adequate temperature, salt concentration [1], any alteration within these parameters affects the changes produced by the enzymes and the subsequent action of the various microorganisms and insects involved in the process.

2.1 Preservative phenomena

Adipocira, also known as saponification, is a change involving the fatty acids present in the tissue, consisting of the breakdown and subsequent hydroxylation of triglycerides, which, as their melting point increases, are transformed into a kind of grayish, rather friable wax [7].

The mummification process is characterized by the desiccation of tissues in which the whole body, segments of it, or different types of tissues are maintained in a state of apparent preservation, stopping the characteristic processes occurring in the decomposition phenomena [8]. This process can occur in two ways: spontaneous or natural and anthropogenic or artificial. In natural mummification, circumstances such as environmental conditions stand out: certain types of climates and soil characteristics in relation to the concentration of various chemical components such as salts, which would favor natural mummification. On the other hand, the artificial mummification process involves a series of procedures carried out on the corpse such as the addition of preservative chemicals, via arterial perfusion or immersion, to preserve the body for as long as possible by means of the technique known as cadaveric preservation or embalming [9].

2.2 Mechanisms of mummification

Historically, the need has arisen to carry out studies with mummified bodies or tissues, from a medicolegal point of view to the study of the sociocultural characteristics of individuals [8]. As the mechanisms of mummification are varied and there are numerous factors that affect or influence the process in one way or another, to better understand them, it is necessary to categorize them [8].

The types of mummification can be classified as follows:

1. Artificial (anthropogenic) mummification.

2. Natural (spontaneous) mummification.

3. Augmented spontaneous mummification.

4. Indeterminate mummification.

The mechanisms of spontaneous mummification are the most important, since from the histopathological point of view, the changes that occur in tissues are related to environmental characteristics [8].

As mentioned above, for the enzymatic degradative activity of the cell and microorganisms to occur, tissues present a large amount of water, oxygen, and other substrates in their composition; therefore, a rapid dehydration of the tissue allows a decrease in the rate of degradation, due to little or no enzymatic activity. Environmental factors such as high temperature and humidity generate a rapid decomposition; on the contrary, a low environmental humidity produces a slow decomposition due to the evaporation of moisture from the corpse, which partially prevents the phenomena of autolysis and putrefaction [10]. The saline concentration of the soil or the environment favors desiccation, since it generates a process of cellular dehydration by osmosis, both in the tissue and in the microorganisms [11].

2.3 Desiccation

Desiccation is the spontaneous preservation process characteristic of mummification, which corresponds to the dehydration of tissues. The tissue loses water due to different factors, especially environmental ones, the most influential as previously mentioned correspond to extremely hot and dry climates, which favor natural mummification; an example of this is the high heat of desert climates that generates the rapid loss of water in soft tissues [1]. Environments with good ventilation or dry air currents would also allow mummification [12]. Another type of desiccation is that caused by freezing, since in extremely cold environments, the low temperature favors mummification mechanisms, due to the decrease in enzymatic activity [13]. Desiccation by chemical factors, such as different types of salts, favors mummification due to dehydration by water outflow or osmosis, in addition to the fact that the high salt concentration alkalinizes the initial acidic environment in which enzymes develop their activity, which causes a decrease in the enzymatic activity of the cells [8]. Another important chemical factor is the concentration of heavy metals in the soil, such as arsenic, mercury, and copper, among others, which completely inactivate the enzymatic action in the degradative processes [14].

2.4 Current embalming methods

Throughout history, there have been several methods of cadaveric preservation; these have varied, from evisceration and use of different components, such as spices, resins, and some types of salts to fill the cavities, to contemporary methods that use different chemical components such as alcohol, formaldehyde, and glycerin, among others in a mixture that is perfused to the corpse by arterial route, or the sample is left in immersion [9]. It should be noted that this process is used for funerary purposes to delay the degradative processes or for academic purposes of a more permanent preservation, for teaching purposes in Normal Anatomy, Pathology, or Forensic Medicine.

2.5 Recovery and rehydration

The macroscopic and microscopic study of tissues in initial stages of decomposition and mummified tissues should be very rigorous, and it should be considered that the expectations regarding the process cannot be very high, since each tissue presents its own characteristics, related to the cause of death, form of maintenance, conservation, and environmental conditions, among others, which are relevant factors that generate characteristic results for each sample, after recovery or rehydration.

As decomposed tissues are friable and mummified tissues are hard and brittle, both are very difficult to handle, process, and analyze. The study at the macroscopic level does not provide much evidence for the analysis of lesions or other characteristics, and on the microscopic aspect, due to routine histopathological processing, the results can be very variable. For these reasons, it is of the utmost importance to have recovery and rehydration protocols that give relatively adequate results, that is, that provide a morphology in which tissue characteristics can be identified to guide the recognition and analysis of forensic medical aspects, as elements of identification of the individual or lesions.

2.6 Rehydration solutions

Most of the rehydration solutions that recover tissues have as main components alcohol, formaldehyde and a salt that provides an adequate osmolarity. The alcohol used corresponds in most cases to ethanol in concentrations between 70° and 95° and is used for its diffusion capacity in the tissue, added to its fixative properties that are complemented with the fixative properties of formaldehyde. Some authors mention that the use of formaldehyde is irrelevant and remove it from their solutions [15]. Other authors mention the importance of using a medium similar in pH and osmolarity in the rehydrating solution, mixing ethanol with some buffer [16]. Within the classification of alcohol-formaldehyde solutions, mention should be made of Sandison's solution, which stands out for providing good results in rehydration protocols and for being one of the most widely used [17].

Consequently, over time, a series of studies have attempted to determine the solution that allows optimal rehydration; however, the quality of the tissue, the type of tissue, and the conditions under which the tissue degrades and/or mummifies, among multiple other factors establish that the vast majority of the methods used provide different results when considering the main criteria that are evaluated in the tissue, such as its morphology and structural integrity, from the point of view of the identification of tissue and cellular structures [17].

Objectively, a rehydration solution would give the best results if it tried to emulate the usual conditions in which living tissue is found. Because of this, human serum began to be used due to its similarity to the internal environment in which the cells are found; however, its use began to be discouraged due to the presumption that in the microscopic analysis, it could generate cross-reactions in the immunohistochemical analysis, generating a nonspecific background that does not provide adequate information on certain tissue components. Therefore, variations to this methodology have been proposed, such as the use of heat-inactivated serum, which provides a rehydration that gives adequate immunohistochemical results [18].

One of the revolutions in rehydration corresponded to the use of commercial fabric softeners in rehydration protocols [19]. There is a wide range of softeners on the market, and in many cases, their components and concentrations are not detailed; however, most of them contain polyamides, some esters, and surfactant amines, which would give "reorganizing" properties to the tissue, giving good results in tissues of high hardness such as fibrocartilage [17].

In the recovery and rehydration process, the fundamental aspect corresponds to the concentration of the solutions, since the solution must be hypotonic, a characteristic that allows it to enter the tissues and cells, reorganizing the remnants that are altered, either by degradation or by mummification.

Another relevant point is the time in which the samples remain in the recovery or rehydrating solution; the time is determined in relation to the characteristics of the tissue to be recovered, whether it is very degraded or very dehydrated, the times can vary, being this a determining step in the processing. Excessive rehydration generates tissue rupture and cell lysis; on the contrary, deficient rehydration impairs the subsequent steps in tissue analysis [20].

An adequate recovery and rehydration can provide adequate results in the cellular and tissue structure, but it must be considered that there are variations due to the multiple circumstances to which the tissues were subjected.

The purpose of these procedures is not only to carry out studies on mummified tissues; however, an important field is the forensic aspect and postmortem analysis, especially in expertise related to tissue findings or exhumations, which allow to clarify injuries and even the cause of death, as well as the use of rehydrating solutions in the recovery of fingerprints with the subsequent or subsequent identification of individuals [21].

2.7 Results in tissue recovery and rehydration

As a reference, the tissues most commonly used for rehydration procedures correspond to skin and skeletal muscle, since they are usually found with greater availability in the body or body segments, with some degree of decomposition or mummified. Internal organs, due to autolysis and putrefaction processes, usually do not give good results in the recovery procedure [20].

Due to the above, it is important to manage a tissue recovery and rehydration protocol that provides adequate morphological results related to the objective of the study. As mentioned above, the solution should be hypotonic in its composition and preferably use low molecular weight molecules that allow diffusion to the tissues, such as sodium bicarbonate, ammonia solution, sodium chloride, and potassium hydroxide, among others.

It should be noted that a standardized protocol based on times and concentrations depends on the type of sample to be recovered or rehydrated; this is at the discretion of the researchers, since variations in the concentrations can generate a decrease or increase in the immersion times in which the sample is left in the solution. For example, more hardened samples require longer rehydration times.

Despite this, the literature describes times from 18 to 24 hours in the recovery and rehydration protocols [17]. Because of this, it is necessary to perform the procedure with the greatest possible dedication, considering in the first instance the macroscopic aspects of the sample. It should be noted that after recovery or rehydration, the sample should be preserved by fixation according to each investigator's own protocols, suggesting fixation in 10% w/v formaldehyde and/or 10% w/v glycerin.

2.8 Macroscopic results

Next, some macroscopic results in the recovery and rehydration of tissues are presented, using the rehydration solution with standardized times, fundamentally based on the macroscopic changes that the samples had and the color and texture to the touch, when being evaluated in the passage of time subjected to immersion.

Figure 1 shows the sample of a human hand in the initial state of decomposition, in which a dark color is observed, including some larvae in the sample.

Figure 2 shows the same sample after 30 hours, subjected to the immersion recovery process.

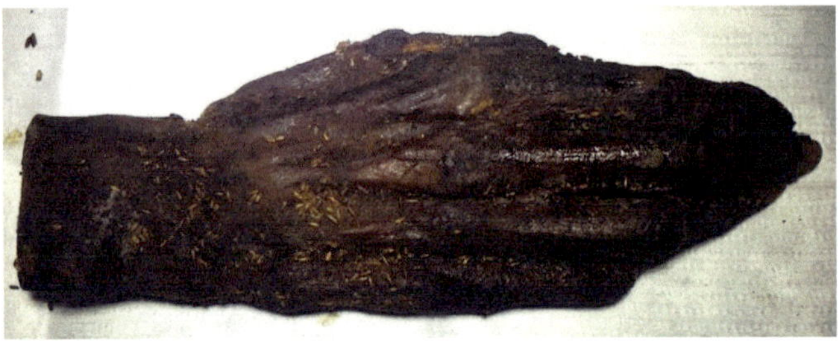

Figure 1.
Dorsal side of the hand in the initial state of decomposition.

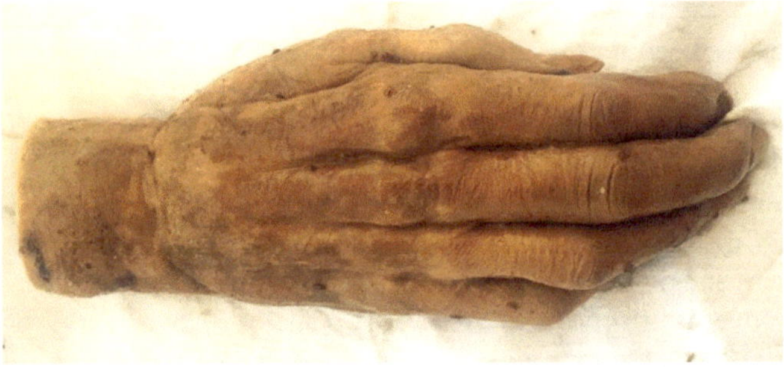

Figure 2.
Dorsal aspect of the hand, after 30 hours of recovery.

Figures 3 and **4** show the sample of a human hand mummified by desiccation; the dried tissues stand out; the texture of these was quite hard and presented a great rigidity.

Figures 5 and **6** show the results of the rehydration process of the sample after 72 hours in immersion. **Figure 7** shows that the protocol allows recovering the flexibility of the sample.

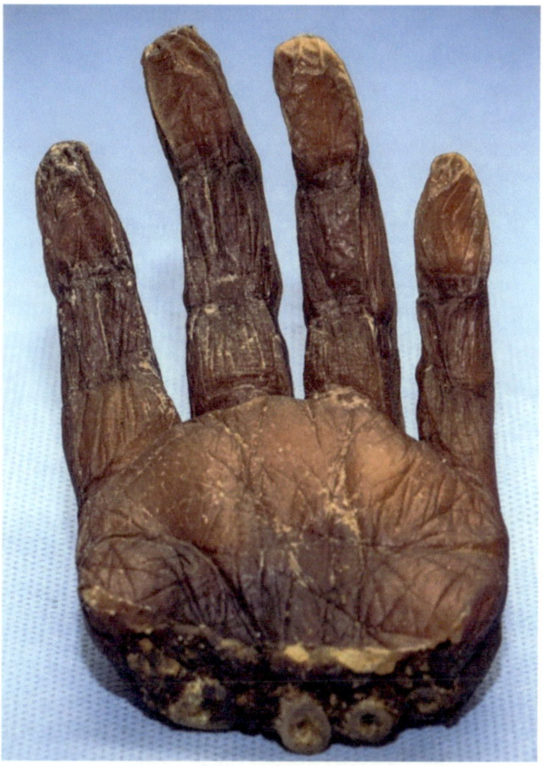

Figure 3.
Palmar side of the hand mummified by desiccation.

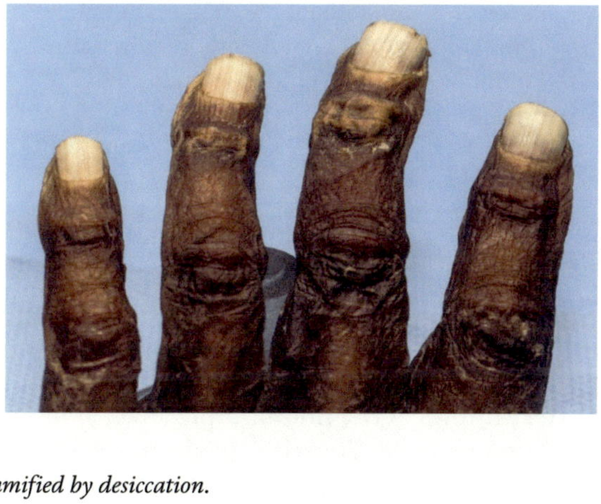

Figure 4.
Dorsum of the hand mummified by desiccation.

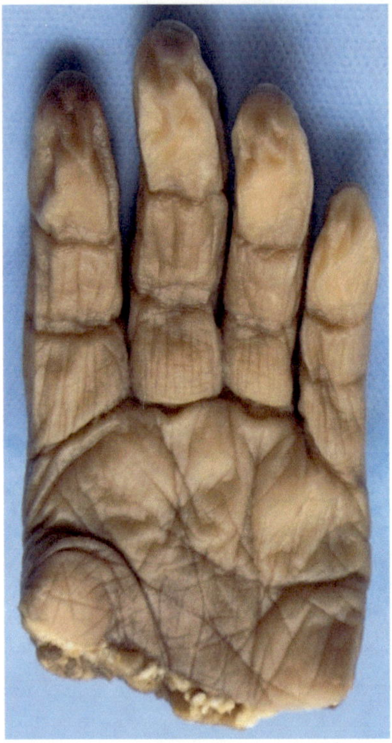

Figure 5.
Palmar side of the hand, after 72 hours of rehydration.

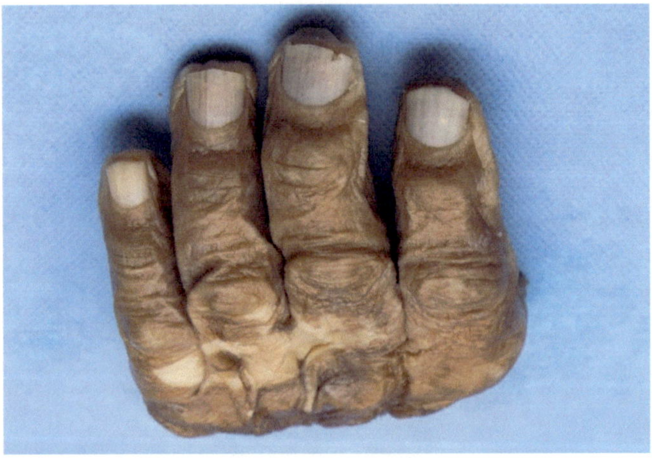

Figure 6.
Dorsum of the hand, after 72 hours of rehydration.

2.9 Microscopic results

For the analysis of the samples at the microscopic level, skin samples were taken from a leg in a state of decomposition **Figure 8**, (red square).

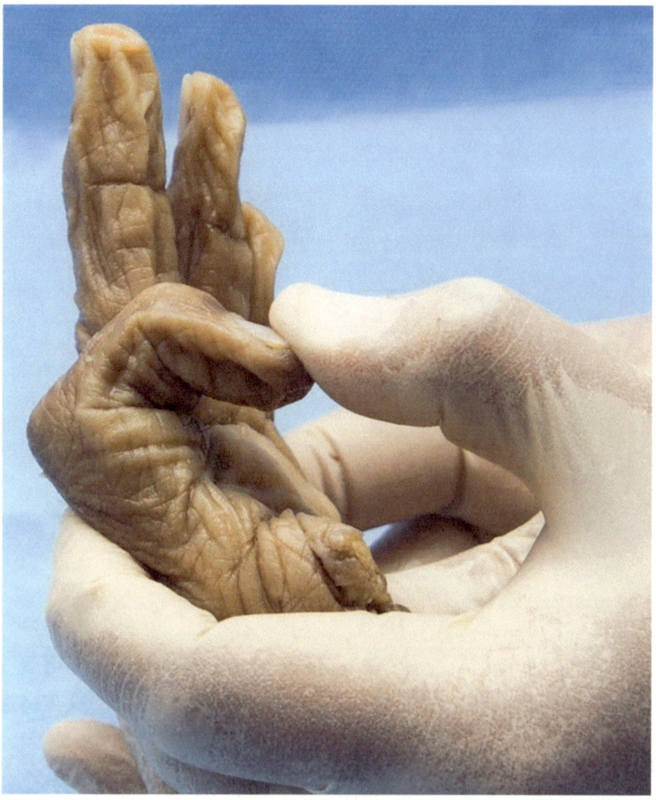

Figure 7.
Recovery of the sample flexibility.

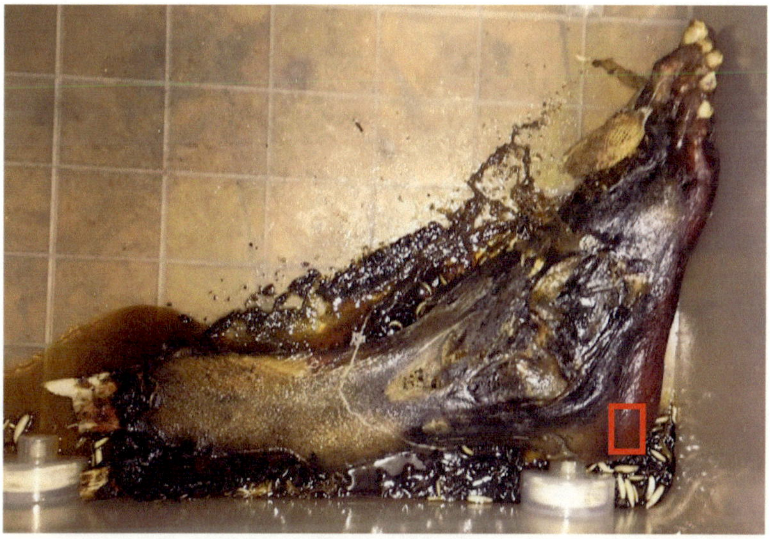

Figure 8.
Decomposing leg, red square corresponds to the area where the sample was taken.

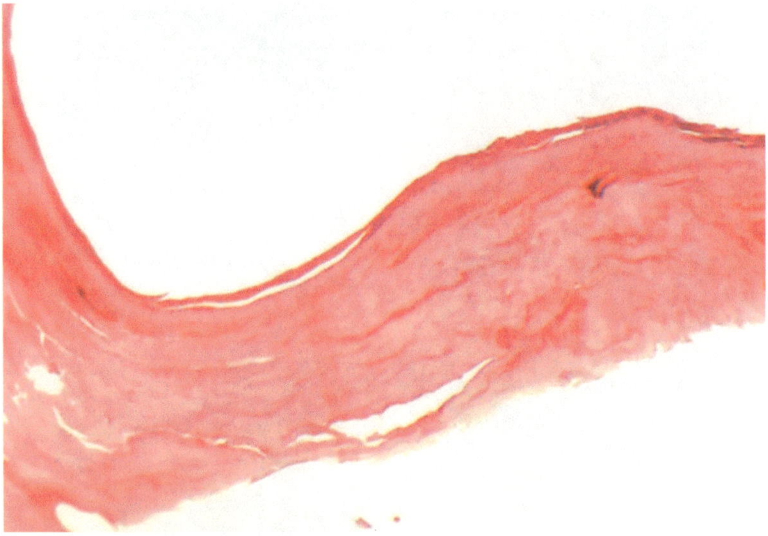

Figure 9.
Skin sample without rehydration protocol, H/E, 100×.

Two skin samples were taken, one sample that was not subjected to the recovery process (**Figure 9**), and one sample that was subjected to the recovery process for 25 hours (**Figure 10**). Both samples were submitted to the routine histotechnical process. The samples were stained with Hematoxylin–Eosin. **Figure 9** shows the skin without recovery, as a compact cut, where the layers of the skin are not evident. On the other hand, **Figure 10** shows a tissue in which the skin layers are differentiated.

To differentiate the tissue components of the skin, such as the dermis and epidermis. Both samples were stained with Van Gieson's trichrome technique. **Figure 11** shows a sample that was not subjected to the rehydration process, which despite

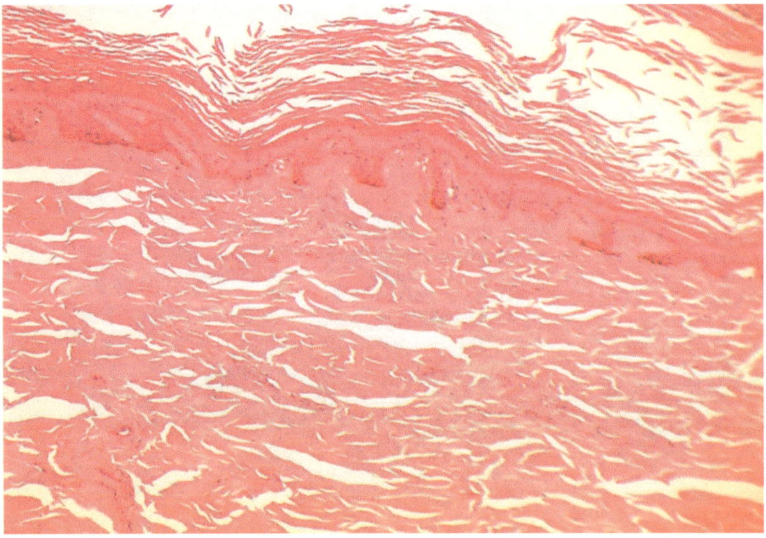

Figure 10.
Skin sample subjected to H/E rehydration protocol, 100×.

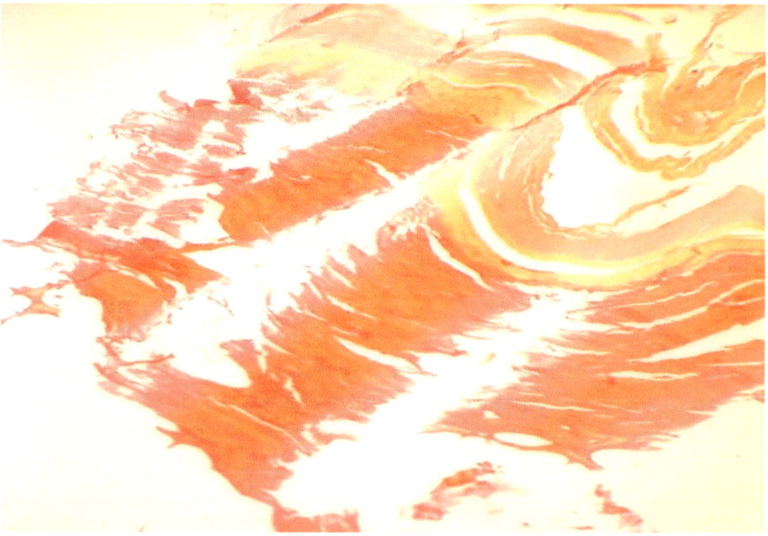

Figure 11.
Skin sample without rehydration protocol, Van Gieson, 100×.

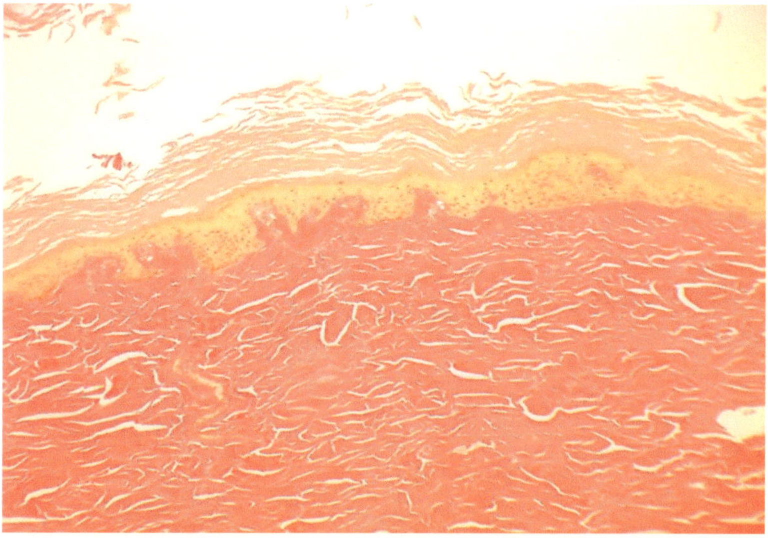

Figure 12.
Skin sample subjected to rehydration protocol, Van Gieson, 100×.

having differentiation of the tissue components, is very disintegrated. **Figure 12** shows the sample subjected to the rehydration process. Here the layers of the skin can be seen, differentiating the epidermis from the connective tissue of the dermis.

3. Conclusion

The study of tissues in the initial state of decomposition or mummified represents a challenge in postmortem analysis, since it is a complex subject due to the processes that allow the tissue to reach these states. This process is influenced by multiple factors, among which the characteristics of the type of tissue, as well as environmental factors, stand out.

The objective of the study and the expectations regarding the process of recovery and rehydration of the tissues is the first factor that must be considered, since it depends on the condition of the tissue and a previous evaluation must be made to determine concentrations and recovery time in the immersion solution. Considering from this aspect that not all tissues can be submitted to the recovery process, since it depends on the conditions in which the sample is found, tissues in certain states of decomposition or mummified can degrade due to an abrupt entrance of the rehydrating solution, which would alter the objective of the study in an important way.

There are many areas where these techniques can be used, one example is in post-mortem analysis. From a macroscopic point of view, it can provide information related to identification elements such as tattoos, marks, scars, lesions, and so forth. And in the microscopic field related to Forensic Pathology, it can provide information on vital or postmortem injuries and pathological conditions among other factors that have generated alterations in the tissue.

Author details

William Aguilar-Navarro* and Carmen Cerda-Aguilar
University of Chile, Santiago, Chile

*Address all correspondence to: waguilar@uchile.cl

References

[1] Galloway A, Birkby W, Jones A, Henry T, Parks B. Decay rates of human remains in an arid environment. Journal of Forensic Sciences. 1989;**34**(3):607-616

[2] Aufderheide A. Soft tissue taphonomy: A paleopathology perspective. International Journal of Paleopathology. 2011;**1**:75-80

[3] Dent B, Forbes S, Stuart B. Review of human decomposition process in soil. Environmental Geology. 2004;**45**:576-585

[4] Fiedler S. Decomposition of buried corpses, with special reference to the formation of adipocere. Die Naturuissenschafter. 2003;**90**:291-300

[5] Vass A, Barshick S, Sega G, Caton J, Skeen J, Love J, et al. Decomposition chemistry of human remains: A new methodology for determining the postmortem interval of human remains. Journal of Forensic Sciences. 2002;**47**(3):542-553

[6] Campobasso CP, Di Vella G, Introna F. Factors affecting decomposition and Diptera colonization. Forensic Sciece International. 2001;**120**(1-2):18-27

[7] Schoenen D, Schoenen H. Adipocere formation--the result of insufficient microbial degradation. Forensic Science International. 2013;**226**:301-306

[8] Aufderheide A. Chapter 3 mechanisms of mummification. In: The Scientific Study of Mummies. Cambridge: Cambridge University Press; 2003. pp. 41-63

[9] Hanzlick R. Embalming, body preparation, burial, and disinterment. An overview for forensic pathologists. The American Journal of Forensic Medicine and Pathology. 1994;**15**(2):122-131

[10] Mann R, Bass W, Meadows L. Time since death and decomposition of the human body: Variables and observations in case and experimental field studies. Journal of Forensic Sciences. 1990;**35**:103-111

[11] Berkeley R, Campbell R. Nutrition, and the influence of environmental factors on microbial activities. In: Hawker LE, Linton AH, editors. Microorganisms Function, Form, and Environment. 2nd ed. Baltimore, Maryland: University Park Press; 1979. pp. 69-82

[12] Kaufmann B. Mummification in the middle ages. In: Spindler K et al, editors. Human Mummies a Global Survey of Their Status and the Techniques of Conservation. 1st ed. Vienna: Springer Vienna; 1996. pp. 231-248

[13] Spindler K, Wilfing H, et al. Human Mummies: A Global Survey of their Status and the Techniques of Conservation. New York: Springer-Verlag, Wien; 1996

[14] Arriaza B. Arseniasis as an environmental hypothetical explanation for the origin of the oldest artificial mummification practice in the world. Revista de Antropología Chilena. 2005;**37**:255-260

[15] Simmandl E. A contribution to the histology of the skin and of the muscle of an egyptian mummy. L'Anthropologie. 1928;**6**:56

[16] Fechner G, Petkovits T, Brinkmann B. Morphologische Identifizierung mumifizierter

Gewebsspuren. Archiv für Kriminologie. 1988;**182**:154-158

[17] Mekota A, Vermehren M. Determination of optimal rehydration, fixation, and staining methods for histological and immunohistochemical analysis of mummified soft tissues. Biotechnic & Histochemistry. 2005;**80**(1):7-13

[18] Herman B. A simple method for softening and rehydration of dried and mummified tissues. Paleopath News. 1982;**39**:10

[19] Turner P, Holtom D. The use of a fabric softener in the reconstitution of mummified tissue prior to paraffin wax sectioning for light microscopical examination. Stain Technology. 1981;**56**:35-38

[20] Fulcheri E, Ventura L. Rileggendo tra antiche e nuove ricette per dare freschezza ai tessuti mummificati o disseccati. Pathologica. 2001;**93**:700-706

[21] Schmidt C, Nawrocki S, Williamson M, Marlin D. Obtaining fingerprints from mummified fingers: A method for tissue rehydration adapted from the archeological literature. Journal of Forensic Science. 2000;**45**(4):874-875

Chapter 5

Samples Used in Molecular Autopsy: An Update

Simone Grassi, Estefanía Martínez-Barrios, Francesca Cazzato, Sergio Cesar, María Luisa Ortega-Sánchez, Eneko Barberia, Elena Arbelo, Antonio Oliva, Georgia Sarquella-Brugada and Oscar Campuzano

Abstract

Molecular autopsy makes it possible to identify the genetic alteration responsible for an inherited arrhythmogenic disease, main suspected cause of sudden death in cases that remain unexplained after a complete medico-legal autopsy. By using next-generation sequencing technology, a massive genetic study can be carried out that identifies a rare variant classified as potentially pathogenic in up to 25% of sudden death cases in the young population. To carry out a post-mortem genetic study, it is necessary to have samples in suitable conservation conditions. Our chapter focuses on the type of samples that are used today in massively parallel genetic analyses.

Keywords: samples, molecular autopsy, genetics, tissue, paraffin, blood

1. Introduction

Currently, in nearly 5% of all cases after comprehensive forensic autopsy no definite cause of death is found, allowing for the definition of "negative autopsy" [1]. When autopsy fails to find the cause of decease, sudden death can be called "unexplained" (SUD) [2]. In SUD cases, especially in those younger than 35 years, inherited arrhythmogenic syndrome (IAS), are frequent cause of death and thus, sudden cardiac death (SCD) should always be suspected [3]. All IAS are of genetic origin and therefore, family members can be carriers of pathogenic genetic alterations, and in consequence, be at risk for SUD. The first manifestation of any of IAS may be a lethal arrhythmogenic episode, highlighting early identification of genetic carriers and allowing the adoption of preventive personalized therapeutic measures [4]. In 2001, a post-mortem genetic analysis or post-mortem molecular analysis (also called "molecular autopsy") was firstly proposed [5] as a fundamental tool in order to unravel the genetic origin of an IAS as cause of SUD [2]. To date, molecular autopsy has become a complement to autopsies process in the current forensic area. Molecular autopsy has been shown to be a reliable diagnostic tool during a comprehensive forensic investigation of SUDs and may have important implications for the

IntechOpen

first-degree relatives of the victim leading to further analyses to predict and prevent the risk of life-threatening events [6].

2. Genetic analysis

First genetic approach in molecular autopsy was Sanger technology which has played a significant role allowing the identification of the first genes associated with IAS related to SCD. Although, the Sanger sequencing technique has played an important role in the history of molecular genetics and has been very useful in the study of SCD for many years, at present, its use in clinical practice has been reduced [7]. For years, Sanger sequencing was the gold standard for investigating SUD cases until it was replaced by second-generation high-throughput techniques, called Next generation sequencing (NGS) [8]. This is due to the fact that Sanger technology only allows the study of a limited number of genes and at a high cost, compared to massive next-generation sequencing techniques. However, it remains the gold standard technique for variant confirmation, especially for small deletions and insertions. Nowadays available NGS technologies allow a rapid and cost-effective genetic analysis of numerous genes (even whole exome -WES- and genome -WGS- sequencing). NGS has enabled the identification of more than 2400 new disease-associated genes and more than 150 new genetic diseases [9].

Finally, third-generation sequencing technologies, also known as single-molecule sequencing, allow for the direct sequencing of single DNA molecules without the need for amplification or fragmentation. Although this technology promises to improve the range of detection of causal variants in a wide range of pathologies, since it has some advantages such as the possibility of studying structural variants and repetitive elements, its implementation in clinical practice has not yet materialized. It is partly due to certain limitations such as the high cost compared to NGS, the need for a more complex bioinformatics analysis, and perhaps the most important limitation in our field, the fact that it requires fresh material to obtain ultralong DNA of high molecular weight, which can be a great challenge in post-mortem analysis [10, 11].

3. NGS applicability to SUD

The routinary genetic study carried out using NGS technology in SUD consist of analyzing the main genes currently associated with IAS, either by amplification and sequencing of gene panels, or by performing WES and subsequent filtering of the genes of interest [12–14]. The number of genes analyzed increase as progress is made in the field of IAS [15]. In young population, molecular autopsy using NGS reveals a definite pathogenic genetic alteration responsible of an IAS in near 20% of cases [16–22]. It is important to remark that genetic alterations identified in IAS are genetic defects in ion channels expressed in heart as well as in brain, therefore being the main cause of sudden death episodes during epilepsy (Sudden Unexpected Death in Epilepsy, SUDEP) [23–25].

After molecular autopsy with a positive genetic diagnosis, due to other family members could harbor the same genetic variant and, thus at risk of IAS, a clinical translation of genetic results should be performed [4]. In such cases, first-degree relatives of a SUD victim should undergo a multidisciplinary evaluation including clinical examination and genetic analysis [6, 26]. To date, main challenge in clinical translation of genetic data is the interpretation of large part of variants identified, remaining of unknown significance (VUS). Firstly, this is due to the stricter classification provided by the American College of Medical Genetics (ACMG) [27]. Moreover, either variants are found in genes with no definite association with any of IAS or available data does not allow a deleterious role of a variant to be assigned. Despite this fact, current clinical guidelines recommend molecular autopsy in SUD cases when the victim is young (< 50 years of age) and/or the circumstances of death and/or the family history support an IAS as the most plausible cause of SUD [4, 6, 28, 29].

4. Samples

Collection of samples for molecular autopsy is a crucial step in the forensic analysis of SUD and is recommended by several guidelines [6, 30]. Suitable sampling in terms of site and of timing is crucial also because of the risk of low-template DNA, i.e., inadequate quality and/or quantity of extracted DNA. Indeed, in IAS, up to 40% of samples are not collected adequately for post-mortem genetic study preventing an appropriate analysis [31]. In an exploratory study, fresh blood and frozen blood were reported as the most common types of post mortem samples. In addition, fresh blood and frozen blood had the highest number of successful DNA extractions, but blood spot cards, frozen liver, and frozen heart tissue were also reported to have successful DNA extractions [32]. Recently, a consensus focused on post-mortem study of SCD cases was published, recommending blood as optimal sample for molecular autopsy despite other kind of samples can be also used if appropriate collection and storage, such as fresh/frozen tissues or formalin-fixed and paraffin-embedded (FFPE) tissues [14].

4.1 Blood

This is the easier approach to obtain and storage a post-mortem sample in order to perform a molecular autopsy. The sample will be preferably extracted from the subclavian vasculature by puncture prior to opening the thoracic cavity. If not possible, the thoracic and abdominal cavities will be opened, removing the visceral blockage and puncturing the right atrium afterwards for blood collection [33]. It is recommended to collect 3–5 ml of peripheral or intracardiac blood less than 48 hours post-mortem in Ethylene Diamine Tetra Acetic acid (EDTA) tubes (**Figures 1** and **2A**). If sample is collected more than 48 hours post-mortem, the degradation of DNA increases progressively despite conservation of body at cold temperature. This degradation may impede a proper DNA extraction and NGS analysis. EDTA tubs should be also store at cold temperature (4–8°C) but if DNA will be extracted during first 48 hours after collection, tubes can be retained at room temperature (no more than 20°C) [34]. If DNA extraction will be programmed more than 2 days after collection, it is highly recommended store tubes at 4°C (maximum 2–4 weeks) [34]. More than one month after extraction, DNA may be progressively degraded, so freezing at a minimum of −20 to −80°C is recommended [14, 35]. However, it is important to note that freezing the EDTA tube should be avoided as much as possible, as the freezing and thawing process damages the DNA structure. In this situation, and in order to preserve DNA integrity, thawing process should be performed progressively (−20 to 4–8°C for at least 1–2 days, and then to room temperature). DNA extraction should be performed

Blood	***Dried blood spot (DBS)***	***Fresh/frozen tissue***	***Saliva***	***Formalin-fixed and paraffin-embedded***
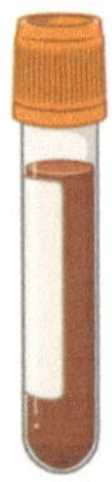	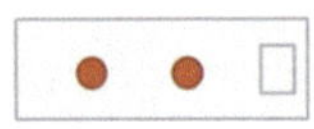	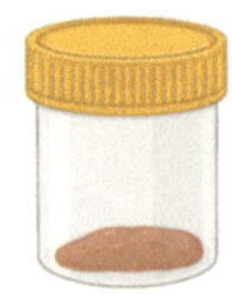	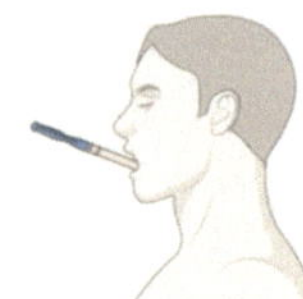	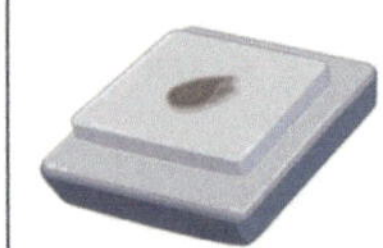
• 4-8°C (max. 48h) • 4°C (max. 2-4 weeks) • -20°C (more than one month)	• -4°C- room temperature (max. 2 weeks). • -20°C (more than 2 weeks).	• 4-8°C (max. 12h). • -20-80°C (more than 12h)	• 37 °C (max. 18 months)	• 37°C (many years)

Figure 1.
Samples used in molecular autopsy analysis and their conservation methods.

at routine room temperature in laboratories (around 15°C). This is the optimal protocol to avoid a rapid DNA degradation, which prevents a proper NGS analysis.

4.2 Dried blood spot (DBS)

Most NGS analyses are performed using EDTA-anticoagulated peripheral blood, because of the high quality of DNA extraction obtained from such samples (**Figure 1**). However, collecting, transporting and storing blood in some circumstances can represent a challenge. An alternative may be the use of Dried blood spots (DBS), since NGS techniques require only short fragments of DNA for sequencing, which can be obtained with this collection technique [14, 35, 36]. DBS is an inexpensive method that is easy to handle in all conditions and does not require a trained professional for collection [37]. DBS can be storage at ambient temperature for many months and even years but the quality of DNA extracted could be reduced progressively [38]. Although recent studies support a sequencing yield with DNA from DBS samples, similar to that obtained with DNA samples from peripheral blood, both in the detection of single nucleotide variants, insertions and deletions, as well as copy number variants and

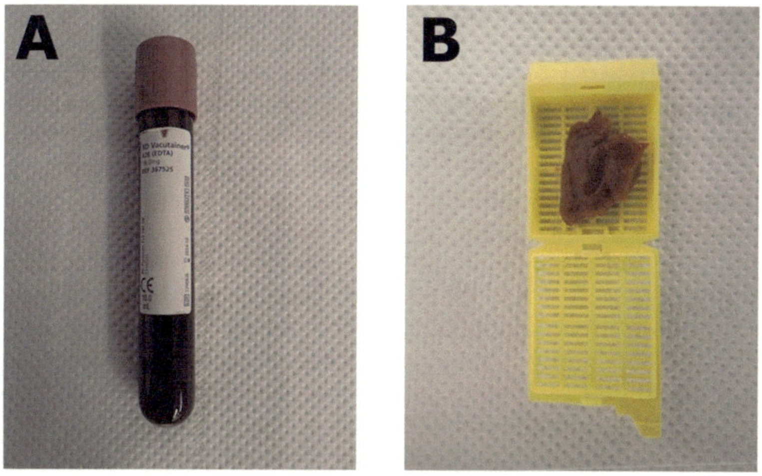

Figure 2.
Real samples mostly used in post-mortem NGS analysis. A. Blood sample. B. Fresh tissue sample.

mitochondrial heteroplasmy, such studies are limited and their throughput in NGS techniques applied to postmortem analysis of SUD has not been confirmed [39–41].

4.3 Fresh/frozen tissue

Fresh tissue samples from cadaver should be collected for post-mortem genetic testing (**Figures 1** and **2B**). The 2020 APHRS/HRS expert consensus statement recommends that samples of heart (especially if SCD is suspected) and at least one spleen/liver/skeletal muscles sample should always be saved [35]. About 5 g of tissue is optimal to perform a quick DNA extraction (no more than 6–12 hours after extraction and retained at 4–8°C) in order to avoid DNA degradation. Focused on SUD and suspected IAS, tissue should be of heart (optimal from ventricular myocardium). If not analyzed in this time period after extraction, the fresh samples should be stored at freezing or ultra-freezing temperatures (−20 to −80°C) [35]. In this situation, defrosting should be carried out progressively (−80 to −20°C, then to 4–8°C for at least 1–2 days, and finally to room temperature) before DNA extraction to avoid degradation, as mentioned for frozen blood. DNA extraction should be performed at routine room temperature in laboratories (around 15°C).

4.4 Saliva

DNA extraction from saliva for high-quality genetic analysis is widely used for living people and many devices are available for the sample collection (**Figure 1**) [42]. It is a widely used sample in the genetic study of many pathologies given the multiple advantages it presents in terms of sample collection, transport and storage. Saliva can be stored at room temperature for up to 18 months without compromising its quality for genetic analysis [43]. Although in forensic genetics buccal swabs are indicated for identification in recent corpses, sampling cadaveric saliva is usually not recommended, since it is technically challenging and can be biased by post-mortem changes. Other samples with the same or lower extraction complexity may yield better quality DNA samples.

4.5 Formalin-fixed and paraffin-embedded (FFPE) tissues

Currently, FFPE tissue samples are processed and stored, as part of routine forensic protocol in order to unravel any tissular alteration (**Figure 1**) [44]. In heart FFPE tissue, several alterations such as inflammatory cell infiltration, myocyte apoptosis or any other alteration may clarify the cause of death. Focused on IAS, tissular alterations may confirm the suspected diagnosis. Sometimes, macroscopic study does not reveal any alteration but FFPE analysis identify alterations such as disarray or fibro-fatty infiltration in myocardium, hallmarks of cardiomyopathies [45]. It is possible to extract DNA from FFPE stored for more than 25 years for molecular analysis [46]. These samples represent a suboptimal material for molecular autopsy as storage in formalin has been shown to damage DNA, which is then variable in both quantity and quality [44, 47].

In order to use FFPE for NGS analysis, protocols of tissue fixation and paraffin embedding usually damages the DNA integrity preventing an adequate NGS study from being performed according the recommended protocols [48]. Tissue samples that were formalin-fixed did not have high rates of successful DNA extraction, which is consistent with evidence found in a past study that showed formalin-fixed samples are unreliable for post mortem genetic testing in cases of sudden unexplained death [32]. DNA from FFPE have been considered error prone and unreliable in comprehensive surveillance of SUD-associated genes. Given these shortcomings, the standard autopsy for SUD should include archiving EDTA-preserved blood or frozen tissue to facilitate post mortem genetic testing [49].

However, several studies have been carried out obtaining proper DNA from FFPE heart tissue in IAS but with a wide range of technical variables preventing a standardized use of FFPE for a comprehensive NGS analysis [50, 51]. In order to solve this limitation, in last years, adapting protocols and special kits focused on DNA extraction from FFPE samples has been developed, helping to use this kind of samples, especially in old cases if no other sample available.

5. Ethics considerations

Although in some countries it is not necessary to have a specific and express consent to perform a genetic analysis on the sample of a deceased person, current legislation must be taken into account before performing a molecular autopsy. When identifying a genetic alteration responsible for the pathology or if the results of the studies are of interest to other members of the deceased's family, it is important to take into account ethical concepts to preserve the privacy and protection of the family members' data, as well as the impact on the health of the individuals who may be at risk. In the case of minors or individuals with intellectual disabilities, the parents or guardians/legal representatives are the ones who must make the decision for them. Communication of the results of genetic testing and autopsy to the family should ideally be performed by a multidisciplinary team composed of cardiologists and genetic counselors specialized in cardiovascular genetics at a medical center, in the context of genetic counseling [14].

6. Conclusions

Finding the cause of the death in SUD cases should be considered a public health priority since, especially in young population, these events are mainly due to IAS.

The current standard techniques for postmortem molecular analysis are those focused on panels of known SUD-associated genes, both because it allows the analysis of a large number of genes at low cost, and because it requires a small amount of DNA obtained from a wide variety of samples for analysis. Sampling is a crucial step in molecular autopsy to avoid the risk of low-template DNA and thus to maximize DNA yield. Post-mortem blood and fresh or frozen highly vascularized tissues are optimal sources of DNA, while the recourse to FFPE tissues should be reserved when other strategies are not feasible, since the risk of low-template DNA.

Acknowledgement/funding

This work was supported by Obra Social "La Caixa Foundation" (LCF/PR/GN19/50320002). Co-funded by Instituto de Salud Carlos III (FIS PI21/00094). CIBERCV is an initiative of the ISCIII, Spanish Ministry of Economy and Competitiveness. Funders had no role in study design, data collection, data analysis, interpretation, or writing of the report.

Conflict of interest

All authors have reported that they have no relationships relevant to the contents of this paper to disclose.

Author details

Simone Grassi[1†], Estefanía Martínez-Barrios[2,3,4†], Francesca Cazzato[5], Sergio Cesar[2,3,4], María Luisa Ortega-Sánchez[6,7], Eneko Barberia[6,8], Elena Arbelo[3,9,10,11], Antonio Oliva[5], Georgia Sarquella-Brugada[2,3,4,12*‡] and Oscar Campuzano[11,12,13*‡]

1 Department of Health Sciences, Section of Forensic Medical Sciences, University of Florence, Florence Italy

2 Pediatric Arrhythmias, Inherited Cardiac Diseases and Sudden Death Unit, Cardiology Department, Sant Joan, Spain

3 European Reference Network for Rare, Low Prevalence and Complex Diseases of the Heart (ERN GUARD-Heart), Amsterdam, The Netherlands

4 Arrítmies Pediàtriques, Cardiologia Genètica i Mort Sobtada, Malalties Cardiovasculars en el Desenvolupament, Institut de Recerca Sant Joan de Déu, Esplugues de Llobregat, Barcelona, Catalonia, Spain

5 Section Legal Medicine, Institute of Public Health, Catholic University, Rome, Italy

6 Forensic Pathology Department, Institut de Medicina Legal i Ciències Forenses de Catalunya (IMLCFC), Barcelona, Spain

7 School of Medicine, Universitat Autònoma de Barcelona, Cerdanyola del Vallés, Spain

8 School of Medicine and Health Sciences, Universitat Rovira i Virgili, Reus, Spain

9 IDIBAPS, Institut d'Investigació August Pi I Sunyer, Spain

10 Arrhythmia Section, Cardiology Department, Hospital Clínic, Universitat de Barcelona, Barcelona, Spain

11 Centro de Investigación Biomédica en Red. Enfermedades Cardiovasculares, Madrid, Spain

12 Medical Science Department, School of Medicine, University of Girona, Girona, Spain

13 Cardiovascular Genetics Center, University of Girona-IDIBGI, Girona, Spain

*Address all correspondence to: georgia@brugada.org and oscar@brugada.org

† These authors contributed equally.

‡Both equally contributed as co-senior authors.

References

[1] Lawler W. The negative coroner's necropsy: A personal approach and consideration of difficulties. Journal of Clinical Pathology. 1990;**43**(12):977-980

[2] Basso C, Aguilera B, Banner J, Cohle S, d'Amati G, de Gouveia RH, et al. Guidelines for autopsy investigation of sudden cardiac death: 2017 update from the Association for European Cardiovascular Pathology. Virchows Archiv. 2017;**471**(6):691-705

[3] Oliva A, Flores J, Merigioli S, LeDuc L, Benito B, Partemi S, et al. Autopsy investigation and Bayesian approach to coronary artery disease in victims of motor-vehicle accidents. Atherosclerosis. 2011;**218**(1):28-32

[4] Wilde AAM, Semsarian C, Marquez MF, Sepehri Shamloo A, Ackerman MJ, Ashley EA, et al. European heart rhythm association (EHRA)/heart rhythm society (HRS)/Asia pacific heart rhythm society (APHRS)/Latin American heart rhythm society (LAHRS) expert consensus statement on the state of genetic testing for cardiac diseases. Heart Rhythm. 2022 Jul;**19**(7):e1-e60.

[5] Ackerman MJ, Tester DJ, Driscoll DJ. Molecular autopsy of sudden unexplained death in the young. The American Journal of Forensic Medicine and Pathology. 2001;**22**(2):105-111

[6] Zeppenfeld K, Tfelt-Hansen J, de Riva M, Winkel BG, Behr ER, Blom NA, et al. 2022 ESC guidelines for the management of patients with ventricular arrhythmias and the prevention of sudden cardiac death. European Heart Journal. 2022;**43**(40):3997-4126

[7] Heather JM, Chain B. The sequence of sequencers: The history of sequencing DNA. Genomics. 2016;**107**(1):1-8

[8] Castiglione V, Modena M, Aimo A, Chiti E, Botto N, Vittorini S, et al. Molecular autopsy of sudden cardiac death in the genomics era. Diagnostics (Basel). 2021 Jul 30;**11**(8):1378

[9] Rabbani B, Nakaoka H, Akhondzadeh S, Tekin M, Mahdieh N. Next generation sequencing: Implications in personalized medicine and pharmacogenomics. Molecular BioSystems. 2016;**12**(6):1818-1830

[10] Xiao T, Zhou W. The third generation sequencing: The advanced approach to genetic diseases. Translational Pediatrics. 2020;**9**(2):163-173

[11] van Dijk EL, Jaszczyszyn Y, Naquin D, Thermes C. The third revolution in sequencing technology. Trends in Genetics. 2018;**34**(9):666-681

[12] Alcalde M, Nogue-Navarro L, Tiron C, Fernandez-Falgueras A, Iglesias A, Simon A, et al. Rare variants in genes encoding structural myocyte contribute to a thickened ventricular septum in sudden death population without ventricular alterations. Forensic Science International Genetics. 2022;**58**: 102688

[13] Coll M, Fernandez-Falgueras A, Tiron C, Iglesias A, Buxo M, Simon A, et al. Post-mortem toxicology analysis in a young sudden cardiac death cohort. Forensic Science International Genetics. 2022;**59**:102723

[14] Kelly KL, Lin PT, Basso C, Bois M, Buja LM, Cohle SD, et al. Sudden cardiac death in the young: A consensus statement on recommended practices for cardiac examination by the pathologist from the Society for Cardiovascular Pathology. Cardiovascular Pathology. 2023 Mar-Apr;**63**:107497

[15] Martinez-Barrios E, Grassi S, Brion M, Toro R, Cesar S, Cruzalegui J, et al. Molecular autopsy: Twenty years of post-mortem diagnosis in sudden cardiac death. Frontiers in Medicine. 2023;**10**: 1118585

[16] Campuzano O, Sanchez-Molero O, Allegue C, Coll M, Mademont-Soler I, Selga E, et al. Post-mortem genetic analysis in juvenile cases of sudden cardiac death. Forensic Science International. 2014;**245C**:30-37

[17] Chugh SS, Senashova O, Watts A, Tran PT, Zhou Z, Gong Q, et al. Postmortem molecular screening in unexplained sudden death. Journal of the American College of Cardiology. 2004; **43**(9):1625-1629

[18] Di Paolo M, Luchini D, Bloise R, Priori SG. Postmortem molecular analysis in victims of sudden unexplained death. The American Journal of Forensic Medicine and Pathology. 2004;**25**(2):182-184

[19] Skinner JR, Crawford J, Smith W, Aitken A, Heaven D, Evans CA, et al. Prospective, population-based long QT molecular autopsy study of postmortem negative sudden death in 1 to 40 year olds. Heart Rhythm. 2011;**8**(3):412-419

[20] Winkel BG, Holst AG, Theilade J, Kristensen IB, Thomsen JL, Hansen SH, et al. Sudden unexpected death in infancy in Denmark. Scandinavian Cardiovascular Journal: SCJ. 2011;**45**(1): 14-20

[21] Tester DJ, Ackerman MJ. The molecular autopsy: Should the evaluation continue after the funeral? Pediatric Cardiology. 2012;**33**(3):461-470

[22] Isbister JC, Nowak N, Butters A, Yeates L, Gray B, Sy RW, et al. "Concealed cardiomyopathy" as a cause of previously unexplained sudden cardiac arrest. International Journal of Cardiology. 2021;**324**:96-101

[23] Bagnall RD, Crompton DE, Petrovski S, Lam L, Cutmore C, Garry SI, et al. Exome-based analysis of cardiac arrhythmia, respiratory control, and epilepsy genes in sudden unexpected death in epilepsy. Annals of Neurology. 2016;**79**(4):522-534

[24] Chahal CAA, Salloum MN, Alahdab F, Gottwald JA, Tester DJ, Anwer LA, et al. Systematic review of the genetics of sudden unexpected death in epilepsy: Potential overlap with sudden cardiac death and arrhythmia-related genes. Journal of the American Heart Association. 2020;**9**(1):e012264

[25] Chahal CAA, Tester DJ, Fayyaz AU, Jaliparthy K, Khan NA, Lu D, et al. Confirmation of cause of death via comprehensive autopsy and whole exome molecular sequencing in people with epilepsy and sudden unexpected death. Journal of the American Heart Association. 2021;**10**(23):e021170

[26] Hansen BL, Jacobsen EM, Kjerrumgaard A, Tfelt-Hansen J, Winkel BG, Bundgaard H, et al. Diagnostic yield in victims of sudden cardiac death and their relatives. Europace. 2020;**22**(6):964-971

[27] Richards S, Aziz N, Bale S, Bick D, Das S, Gastier-Foster J, et al. Standards and guidelines for the interpretation of sequence variants: A joint consensus recommendation of the American College of medical genetics and genomics and the Association for molecular pathology. Genetics in Medicine. 2015;**17**(5):405-424

[28] Ackerman MJ, Priori SG, Willems S, Berul C, Brugada R, Calkins H, et al. HRS/EHRA expert consensus statement

on the state of genetic testing for the channelopathies and cardiomyopathies: This document was developed as a partnership between the heart rhythm society (HRS) and the European heart rhythm association (EHRA). Europace. 2011;**13**(8):1077-1109

[29] Priori SG, Blomstrom-Lundqvist C. 2015 European Society of Cardiology Guidelines for the management of patients with ventricular arrhythmias and the prevention of sudden cardiac death summarized by co-chairs. European Heart Journal. 2015;**36**(41): 2757-2759

[30] Stiles MK, Fauchier L, Morillo CA, Wilkoff BL. 2019 HRS/EHRA/APHRS/LAHRS focused update to 2015 expert consensus statement on optimal implantable cardioverter-defibrillator programming and testing. Heart Rhythm. 2020;**17**(1):e220-e228

[31] Williams N, Manderski E, Stewart S, Bao R, Tang Y. Lessons learned from testing cardiac channelopathy and cardiomyopathy genes in individuals who died suddenly: A two-year prospective study in a large medical examiner's office with an in-house molecular genetics laboratory and genetic counseling services. Journal of Genetic Counseling. 2020;**29**(2):293-302

[32] Liu G, MacLeod H, Webster G, McNally EM, O'Neill SM, Dellefave-Castillo L. Genetic counselors' approach to postmortem genetic testing after sudden death: An exploratory study. Academic Forensic Pathology. 2018;**8**(3): 738-751

[33] Singh D, Tiwari RC, Kumar A, Bhute AR, Meshram RP, Dikshit M, et al. A comprehensive review of pathological examination in forensic medicine: Past, present, and future. Cureus. 2022;**14**(3): e22740

[34] Sanchez O, Campuzano O, Fernandez-Falgueras A, Sarquella-Brugada G, Cesar S, Mademont I, et al. Natural and undetermined sudden death: Value of post-mortem genetic investigation. PLoS One. 2016;**11**(12): e0167358

[35] Stiles MK, Wilde AAM, Abrams DJ, Ackerman MJ, Albert CM, Behr ER, et al. 2020 APHRS/HRS expert consensus statement on the investigation of decedents with sudden unexplained death and patients with sudden cardiac arrest, and of their families. Heart Rhythm. 2021;**18**(1):e1-e50

[36] Boemer F, Fasquelle C, d'Otreppe S, Josse C, Dideberg V, Segers K, et al. A next-generation newborn screening pilot study: NGS on dried blood spots detects causal mutations in patients with inherited metabolic diseases. Scientific Reports. 2017;**7**(1):17641

[37] Martial LC, Aarnoutse RE, Schreuder MF, Henriet SS, Bruggemann RJ, Joore MA. Cost evaluation of dried blood spot home sampling as compared to conventional sampling for therapeutic drug monitoring in children. PLoS One. 2016; **11**(12):e0167433

[38] Gruner N, Stambouli O, Ross RS. Dried blood spots–preparing and processing for use in immunoassays and in molecular techniques. Journal of Visualized Experiments. 2015 Mar 13;**97**: 52619

[39] Agrawal P, Katragadda S, Hariharan AK, Raghavendrachar VG, Agarwal A, Dayalu R, et al. Validation of whole genome sequencing from dried blood spots. BMC Medical Genomics. 2021;**14**(1):110

[40] Anderson C, Fry RC, Hartwell H, Kleeberger C, Sandler DP, Nichols HB.

Measurement of mitochondrial DNA copy number in dried blood spots: A pilot study. Mitochondrion. 2021;**56**:35-39

[41] Hendrix MM, Cuthbert CD, Cordovado SK. Assessing the performance of dried-blood-spot DNA extraction methods in next generation sequencing. International Journal of Neonatal Screening. 2020 Jun;**6**(2):36

[42] Goode MR, Cheong SY, Li N, Ray WC, Bartlett CW. Collection and extraction of saliva DNA for next generation sequencing. Journal of Visualized Experiments. 2014 Aug 27;**90**: 51697

[43] Anthonappa RP, King NM, Rabie AB. Evaluation of the long-term storage stability of saliva as a source of human DNA. Clinical Oral Investigations. 2013;**17**(7):1719-1725

[44] Reid KM, Maistry S, Ramesar R, Heathfield LJ. A review of the optimisation of the use of formalin fixed paraffin embedded tissue for molecular analysis in a forensic post-mortem setting. Forensic Science International. 2017;**280**:181-187

[45] Mathieson W, Thomas GA. Why formalin-fixed, paraffin-embedded biospecimens must be used in genomic medicine: An evidence-based review and conclusion. The Journal of Histochemistry and Cytochemistry. 2020;**68**(8):543-552

[46] Lin J, Kennedy SH, Svarovsky T, Rogers J, Kemnitz JW, Xu A, et al. High-quality genomic DNA extraction from formalin-fixed and paraffin-embedded samples deparaffinized using mineral oil. Analytical Biochemistry. 2009;**395**(2): 265-267

[47] Tester DJ, Ackerman MJ. The role of molecular autopsy in unexplained sudden cardiac death. Current Opinion in Cardiology. 2006;**21**(3):166-172

[48] Srinivasan M, Sedmak D, Jewell S. Effect of fixatives and tissue processing on the content and integrity of nucleic acids. The American Journal of Pathology. 2002;**161**(6):1961-1971

[49] Carturan E, Tester DJ, Brost BC, Basso C, Thiene G, Ackerman MJ. Postmortem genetic testing for conventional autopsy-negative sudden unexplained death: An evaluation of different DNA extraction protocols and the feasibility of mutational analysis from archival paraffin-embedded heart tissue. American Journal of Clinical Pathology. 2008;**129**(3):391-397

[50] Baudhuin LM, Leduc C, Train LJ, Avula R, Kluge ML, Kotzer KE, et al. Technical advances for the clinical genomic evaluation of sudden cardiac death: Verification of next-generation sequencing panels for hereditary cardiovascular conditions using formalin-fixed paraffin-embedded tissues and dried blood spots. Circulation. Cardiovascular Genetics. 2017 Dec;**10**(6):e001844

[51] Lin Y, Gryazeva T, Wang D, Zhou B, Um SY, Eng LS, et al. Using postmortem formalin fixed paraffin-embedded tissues for molecular testing of sudden cardiac death: A cautionary tale of utility and limitations. Forensic Science International. 2020;**308**:110177

Chapter 6

Estimation of Death Time

Melike Erbaş

Abstract

Death time is an issue that is generally requested to be determined by the prosecution offices that request autopsies. The determination of the time of death may be necessary for the heirs to carry out some legal actions and also, from a forensic point of view, to enlighten the case. Although its determination is very important, there is no known scientific method by which the exact time of death can be determined. Generally, the ambient conditions where the corpse is found, the environmental temperatures, and similar factors are evaluated, and the time interval is estimated by considering these factors according to the level of algor mortis, livor mortis, rigor mortis, signs of decomposition or skeletonization. The estimated death time is then reflected in the autopsy report. In this section, we aim to explain in detail how we make these estimations according to the time intervals and environmental conditions, as well as to review the literature in this area.

Keywords: postmortem changes, stages of decomposition, postmortem interval, death time estimation, postmortem examination

1. Introduction

Today, there is no method that can be used alone in the determination of the time of death [1]. It is noteworthy that most of the proposed methods do not have a standardized procedure [1, 2]. Therefore, the term "time of death" should be avoided even if all factors are taken into account [3]. However, it is possible to determine the approximate duration of death as "interval" [3]. The usage of methods such as algor mortis and electrical stimulation of muscles either as isolated methods or in multi-methodological approaches was introduced as reliable in the estimation of early postmortem intervals (PMI) [4, 5]. Along with the physical methods, the usage of biochemical parameters in combination with other parameters were reported to be beneficial [6]. In the journey of scientific advancements. Degradation of nucleic acids over time stands at the attention-grabbing point in the field of PMI estimation [7, 8]. However, in this chapter, we will be focusing on how to estimate the death time during the postmortem external examination in practice by using the factors as postmortem changes and if present phases of decomposition.

2. Usage of postmortem changes in the estimation of death time

2.1 Usage of algor mortis in the estimation of death time

Postmortem body temperature is considered normal at the time of death. There may not be a significant increase or decrease in natural and rapid deaths and forced deaths in postmortem body temperature [9]. In some cases (such as congestive heart failure, massive bleeding, and secondary shocks), the temperature may be subnormal, and in deaths from infections, pons bleeding, and heart attacks, it may be above normal, and in some cases (septicemia, fulminant infections, etc.), it may continue to increase for a few hours post mortem [10].

The use of postmortem interval determination methods based on body temperature is limited due to their high standard deviations [5, 11]. Although there are many schemes used in dead cooling, none of them is completely reliable, and the most useful of these schemes is the Henssge Normograms, with which the estimated time differs from the real time by 2.8 hours [4].

2.2 Usage of rigor mortis in the estimation of death time

After death, the body muscles first relax, and after this event, which is called primary muscle relaxation, stiffness of muscles becomes visible in about 1–3 hours, which is called rigor mortis [12, 13]. There are also cases where it has been reported that rigor mortis occurs within 15–20 minutes [12–14]. It takes approximately 6–12 hours for the rigor mortis to become visible throughout the body [12–14].

The formation of muscle stiffness depends on the consumption of ATP available after death and the lack of new ATP production. ATP is the main energy source required for muscle contraction [12, 14, 15].

The development of stiffness actually occurs in all muscles at the same time; however, it first appears in smaller muscles such as the jaw muscles, so it is said that rigor mortis starts from small muscles and gradually spreads to the whole body [12]. The onset and duration of dead stiffness are closely related to muscle mass and functional state before death [9]. There are many factors such as ambient temperature, physical activity before death, and so on, which affect the formation of dead stiffness [16]. Therefore, PMI cannot be determined by only looking at the rigor mortis parameter. While interpreting PMI during the onset and end of rigor mortis, symptoms such as cooling of the corpse, condition of dead spots, and decay should be evaluated together [9]. Rigor mortis disappears with decomposition in about 36 hours depending on the ambient conditions, but it can be seen to extend up to 6 days [12, 14]. In very hot environments, it can be seen to disappear within 24 hours [14]. Regarding the determination of rigor mortis and PMI, there are experiments in which Kromprecher measures rigor mortis at certain hours [17]. In the study by Hirakawa et al. with Nuclear Magnetic Resonance Spectroscopy, metabolic changes in the femoral muscle of rats after death were examined, and it was reported that the data obtained showed hourly differences, and these differences were correlated with PMI [17].

2.3 Usage of livor mortis in the estimation of death time

Since circulation stops with death, the vascular system and blood physiology completely change. Components in the blood remain under the influence of gravity due to the cessation and immobility of blood flow [12, 18]. Under these conditions, the plasma and cellular contents precipitate, initially forming a sediment within the vascular system of the corpse [19]. Later, it gradually collects from the vascular system into venules and capillaries near the ground, with the effect of gravity, and over time, dark purple and sometimes light red "livor mortis" occur on the skin parts of the corpse that are close to the ground that do not have pressure on [12, 14]. About 30 minutes after death, dead spots that start to form in a period of about 8–12 hours become fixed according to the body position; in cooler environments, it may take 24–36 hours for the dead spots to become fixed [14]. Livor mortis can be seen until the body completely loses its color due to decay [13].

2.4 Usage of postmortem macroscopic changes in the eye in the estimation of death time

Many methods have been proposed for the estimation of the postmortem interval based on the changes in the eye [15].

About 10 minutes after death, the cornea becomes cloudy. If the eyelids remain open in dry weather, the cornea will turn brown in a few hours. At the 10th or 12th hour, the cornea takes on the color of milk. The complete formation of corneal opacity takes the third day [3, 9].

Measurement of intraocular pressure with the tonometer method, which is stated to be used up to the postmortem 6th hour; direct examination of retinal blood vessels with ophthalmoscope; and reflex contraction due to electrical or pharmaceutical stimulation of the iris may be possible in the early postmortem period [15].

It has been observed that reflex contraction can occur with injections of localized catecholamine solution for up to 46 hours following clinical death [15].

Jafaar and Nokes state that eye-related changes such as corneal opacity, retinal vessel segmentation, pupillary reaction, retinal changes, and intraocular pressure changes seen in the postmortem eye can be used in the early detection of PMI [20].

In the study by Kocaturk et al., no relationship was found between pupil diameters and tache noire development and PMI, but it was reported that the rate of corneal clouding was statistically significantly higher ($P < 0.01$) if the postmortem period lasted longer than 8 hours [3].

There is also one other method that uses the excitability of orbicularis oculi found to be reliable, which tests the local contraction and not the whole muscle [4].

2.5 Usage of postmortem stimulations of nerves and muscles

It was first revealed by Professor Luigi Galvani in 1780 that isolated muscle groups can be stimulated by external electrical stimulation [15].

In the determination of PMI, there are subjective and objective measurement methods that examine the changes in skeletal muscles due to postmortem stimulation [4]. Henssge and Madea visually evaluated the muscle response to stimulation and showed that the accuracy of their predictions increased when they used the heat method together with their method [4]. The same researchers also made objective measurements with muscular power conductors placed in the muscle [4]. There are studies in which the peripheral nervous system is also stimulated for the determination of PMI [2].

3. Usage of decomposition in the estimation of death time

Decomposition is a process consisting of autolysis and putrefaction [14]. Autolysis refers to aseptic chemical destruction processes of cells and organs by the help of the intracellular enzymes [14]. Since this is a chemical reaction, it accelerates with temperature, slows down with cold, and stops with freezing [14]. Organs rich in enzymes are autolyzed faster than others [14]. For this reason, the pancreas autolyzes faster than other organs [9].

Bacterial fermentation: After death, the flora in the gastrointestinal tract disperses throughout the body, creating putrefaction [14].

Although the putrefaction varies according to the environmental conditions, it starts with a green color change in the right lower quadrant approximately 36–48 hours after death, and the stage progresses until the skeletonization [9, 14]. There are four phases of decomposition [9].

3.1 First phase of decomposition in the estimation of death time

This period is the beginning of decay; it varies according to ambient conditions. It starts with green coloration of the skin over the cecum, in the right lower quadrant, approximately 36–48 hours after death [9, 10]. Epidermal separations and bulla formations are observed. The gases released as a result of decay are approximately 60–72. It causes the abdomen to begin to swell within hours [14]. The abdomen appears swollen and tense within a week; in conditions where the environment is very hot, swelling can occur in 24 hours, and in very cold environments such as Siberia, putrefaction does not occur even for thousands of years [14]. In common sepsis cases, there are cases where decomposition is observed to accelerate even if the corpse is immediately placed in the refrigerator. It is stated that even if a septic corpse is placed in the refrigerator, it can appear as 5–6 days old within 6–12 hours [14].

In the 3rd and 4th weeks, as the gas and volume increase in the corpse reaches its maximum dimensions, the abdomen bursts [9, 12]. It is thought that this period is completed in approximately 3–4 weeks (1 month) under average conditions of 15–20°C [9, 12].

3.2 Second phase of decomposition in the estimation of death time

With the realization of the explosion in the abdomen, the abdomen and chest wall collapse [9, 12]. All organs look like sacs filled with a mud-like substance (9). After this period, the evaluation of PMI becomes difficult and varies greatly according to conditions [9, 12].

3.3 Third phase of decomposition in the estimation of death time

The liver becoming indistinguishable indicates the beginning of the 3rd period. Muscles gradually begin to separate from their places [9].

3.4 Fourth phase of decomposition in the estimation of death time

When gender becomes indistinguishable from the outside, it is considered to have entered the fourth stage [9]. Depending on the characteristics of the environment in which the corpse is buried, the muscles and joints are separated within a year or two [9, 12]. Although it is not certain, skeletalization is completed in 3–5 years on average, depending on conditions such as soil drainage [9, 12].

Along with the PMI estimation methods made by looking at the postmortem changes in the first hours after death, the stages of decay with the onset of decay and entemological examinations can also be used to determine the time of death in later periods [9, 21].

The use of entomological evidence in the determination of PMI has been known for a long time [9]. Bergeret was the first person to use data on entomofauna in funerals by conducting forensic medical examinations on corpses [21]. After Bergeret, many more comprehensive studies were conducted using the results [21].

There are studies to determine the time elapsed after death and the place where death occurred by examining the changes made by insects on the corpse and the development level of insects [21].

4. Role of biochemistry in the estimation of death time

Studies continue on the use of biochemical analyses in PMI determination [22]. The biochemical parameters studied are hypoxantin, Ca + 2, ammonia in vitreous fluid; K + in the vitreous and cerebrospinal fluid; serum nonprotein nitrogen (NPN); cerebrospinal fluid amino acids; and blood pH [23]. In addition to the convenience of taking blood samples, it is also possible to compare them with pre-mortem values [23]. Another tissue that can be easily sampled and examined postmortem is vitreous fluid [23]. However, since the pre-mortem values are not known, there is no possibility of comparison [23].

Macromolecules and enzymes circulating in tissues with blood circulation, such as glucose, insulin, and alkaline phosphatase, may show quantitative differences between the right and left chambers of the heart as there is no postmortem circulation [23]. For this reason, it is necessary to know the exact place where the blood sample was taken. Taking blood directly from the heart is never recommended, instead, it is generally recommended to use venous samples [23].

Kominato et al. investigated the conversion of a complement factor (C3) to its constituent fragments in the blood for the determination of PMI by immune electrophoresis and suggested that there was a statistically significant correlation between C3 degradation and PMI, and thus, it was reported that PMI could be predicted by looking at the C3 fragmentation rate [24]. Endo et al. measured monoamine metabolites in the cerebrospinal fluid and observed that the concentration of 3–4 dihydroxyphenylacetic acid increased with time after death and reported that it could be used in the determination of PMI [25].

In the study conducted by Doğan et al., it was found that the use of Fe, K, Na, Ca, and Cu elements in rat tissues could be reliable in determining PMI; significant changes were reported in more than one tissue at 4°C and 18 ± 2°C in line with the passing time after death, which needs to be supported by other studies and on other tissues as autopsy tissues [26].

We have recently seen the usage of DNA and RNA degradation in PMI estimation as innovative approaches [27, 28] However, all these studies were evaluated as preliminary that reflects the early phases of the subject where we predominantly see the usage of animal models, containing a lot of uncertainties and depending on various extrinsic and intrinsic factors as environmental conditions, causes of death, and so on [27–31].

5. Estimating the death time during the postmortem examinations

5.1 Why do we try to estimate the death time?

The methods mentioned in the above-mentioned literature generally remain as methods that are not used much in practice at the experimental level [1–3, 22–31]. However, the question of the exact time of death remains on the documents pertaining to the autopsy request made by the prosecution offices.

For every answer to be stated in the autopsy report for this question, it should be emphasized there is no specific scientific method that can give a definite result on this subject. Subjective and empirical estimates can be made about the time of death in the form of intervals, and the estimates obtained in the form of time intervals they receive from us will need to be supported by forensic investigations [1–3, 22–31].

5.2 How do we try to estimate the death time?

5.2.1 Things to be recorded before the postmortem examination

The most important point we should pay attention to in estimating the time of death is that the progression of the postmortem changes that we will use toward decomposition and from decomposition to skeletonization accelerates with higher temperatures, slows down with cold, and stops with freezing [12, 14, 16]. At this point, whether there are personal underlying factors (such as infectious diseases, sepsis, etc.) that may accelerate the progress toward decomposition in the corpse, the air temperatures, and the ambient temperatures where the corpse is located should also be taken into account and recorded [9, 10].

5.2.2 Things to be recorded during the postmortem examination

Postmortem changes should be recorded in particular detail in order to be able to estimate the time of death during the external examination of the cause of death before the autopsy [9, 12, 14]. The items to be recorded can be listed as follows:

1. The temperature of the corpse (rectal temperature) [9].

2. It should be carefully examined and recorded whether rigor mortis, which start to become visible primarily in small joints such as the jaw joint after primary muscle relaxation after death, spread to all muscle groups in the whole body and whether the dead stiffness is resolved. It should be taken into account that dead stiffness may not be observed in joints where the dead stiffness is dissolved by force, and this should not be confused with the onset of decay [9, 12–14].

3. It is important to record whether livor mortis occur or not, and if they do, whether they are fixed or not so that we can estimate the time of death [12–14].

4. If there are signs of decay, at what level they are, whether they are in the form of early signs of decay in the form of greenish discoloration in the abdominal region and the epidermal separations, whether the abdomen is swollen, or whether there is abdominal burst [9, 10, 12, 14].

5. If skeletal remains are brought, whether there are tissue remains on the bones [9, 12].

5.2.3 How do we estimate the time of death after the postmortem examination?

5.2.3.1 If the corpse is still warm?

In cases where the cooling of the dead is not felt yet, and if possible determined that the dead cooling of the corpse has not progressed by rectal measurements, it is important whether livor mortis and rigor mortis have occurred [9, 12, 14].

A still warm corpse without dead stiffness and livor mortis is usually encountered in hospital deaths where the moment of death is known; however, in this case, it would be a more appropriate behavior to check the time of death from the medical records.

If we encounter such a corpse at the crime scene where it is found dead, then it can be said that what we have done is a subjective and empirical estimation and that the death occurred within a maximum of 3 hours backward from the time of the postmortem examination [9, 12–14].

Similarly, in a warm corpse, dead stiffness is not yet observable in large joints, and in cases where livor mortis have just begun to be observed, it can be noted that death can be estimated to have occurred at least 3 hours and at most 6 hours before the time of the postmortem examination, and this given time frame is based on subjective estimations [12–14].

5.2.3.2 If the rigor mortis can be seen throughout the body?

In a corpse where the rigor mortis is visible throughout the body, it is important whether the livor mortis are fixed or not [12–14]. When some pressure is applied to the postmortem lividity, if there is a fading in the area where the pressure is applied or a change of place of the postmortem lividity is observed by changing the position of the corpse, it can be said that the death took place at least 6 hours before the time of the postmortem examination, and the livor mortis become fixed in 24–36 hours in cold environments according to the ambient temperature [9, 12–14].

It should be noted that if there is a corpse with dead stiffness and fixed livor mortis, it can be estimated that the death occurred at least 12 hours before the postmortem examination, and this estimation is not certain [9, 12–14].

5.2.3.3 If there are signs of decomposition?

In a corpse where the solidity of the dead has been dissolved, signs of decay become important. The signs of decay are usually noticed by the greenish discoloration of the lower abdomen and the dissolution of the rigor mortis [9, 10, 14].

Considering that the onset of decomposition in average conditions (at temperatures between 15 and 20 degrees) is 36–48 hours, in a corpse encountered in cold winter conditions and in which the signs of decay are new, death is roughly within a period of at least 48 hours before the postmortem examination [12, 14, 16]. It should be noted that in summer conditions, it can be said that a maximum of 48 hours have passed from when the postmortem examination was performed, and in hot climates and if the corpse has an underlying disease such as sepsis, the signs of decay may begin within 6–12 hours after death [9, 12, 14, 16].

In average conditions, within the first week of death, epidermal separations, together with the swelling of the abdomen and the marbling phenomenon are observed [9, 10, 14]. Although it is noted that swelling in the abdomen can be seen within 24 hours in very hot conditions, it would not be wrong to say that the death occurred within a period of at most 1 week backward from the time of the post-mortem examination in a case where the abdomen is swollen and tense and there are widespread epidermal separations throughout the body [9, 12, 14, 16]. If such a corpse is evaluated at ambient temperatures below 15 degrees, it can be said that at least 1 week has passed since its death [9, 12, 14, 16].

At this point, the expressions "minimum" and "maximum" that we will use while specifying the time period also vary according to the air temperatures and ambient temperatures [9, 12, 14, 16]. For example, it can be said that the death of a corpse with widespread epidermal separations, which we see in 15–20 degrees and hotter conditions; dead stiffness resolved, and extremely tense and swollen abdominal region has occurred within a maximum of 1 week. It can be said that at least 1 week has passed from the time of the death.

It should be noted that when we encounter a corpse with widespread signs of decomposition in the abdomen, at most 1 month has passed since death at temperatures of 15–20 degrees and above, and at least 1 month ago at temperatures below 15 degrees; our estimation is an average estimate [9, 12, 14, 16].

5.2.3.4 Estimation by found bones

In this regard, it may be preferable to perform laboratory tests, if possible, rather than external examination [9]. If we are still asked to make an estimation, an estimation can be made based on the condition of the bone remains. Considering that the skeletonization is completed in 3–5 years on average, the presence of tissue remains suggests that death may have occurred in a time period of at most 3 years, and the completion of the skeletonization without any tissue residues on the bone tissues suggests that at least 3 years have passed since death [9, 12].

5.2.3.5 Estimation by insect activity

The presence of insect eggs in areas such as the nasal and oral cavities does not constitute a very important parameter in determining the time of death, because these eggs can also be seen especially on immobile and debilitated individuals [9, 21].

Time of death can be determined according to the developmental level of insects [9, 21]. This can be achieved by entomological examination of the samples taken during postmortem examination.

Thanks

I would like to thank first my elders in Muğla for being a reason for me to live in Muğla for a while and to my colleagues and the staff of the Muğla directorate of Forensic Medicine Institute, with whom I have worked in harmony for 7 years for their friendship and for the autopsy practice they have added to my adventure in forensic medicine.

Author details

Melike Erbaş
Council of Forensic Medicine, İstanbul, Turkiye

*Address all correspondence to: dr.melikeerbas@gmail.com

References

[1] Henssge C, Madea B. Estimation of the time since death. Forensic Science International. 2007;**165**:182-184

[2] Elmas I, Baslo B, Ertas M, Kaya M. Analysis of gastrocnemius compound muscle action potential in rat after death: Significance for the estimation of early postmortem interval. Forensic Science International. 2001;**116**:125-132

[3] Kocatürk KB, Balcı Y, Bal C. Ölüm zamanı bilinen 200 olguda makroskopik göz bulgularının postmortem interval açısından değerlendirilmesi. Turkiye Klinikleri Journal of Forensic Medicine. 2007;**4**:102-105

[4] Henßge C, Madea B. Estimation of the time since death in the early post-mortem period. Forensic Science International. 2004;**144**:167-175

[5] Nelson EL. Estimation of short-term postmortem interval utilizing core body temperature: A new algorithm. Forensic Science International. 2000;**109**:31-38

[6] Madea B. Is there recent progress in the estimation of the postmortem interval by means of thanatochemistry? Forensic Science International. 2005;**151**:139-149

[7] Di Nunno NR, Costantinides F, Bernasconi P, Bottin C, Melato M. Is flow cytometric evaluation of DNA degradation a reliable method to investigate the early postmortem period? The American Journal of Forensic Medicine and Pathology. 1998;**19**(1):50-53

[8] Marchuk L, Sciore P, Reno C, Frank CB, Hart DA. Postmortem stability of total RNA isolated from rabbit ligament, tendon and cartilage. Biochimica et Biophysica Acta. 1998;**1379**:171-177

[9] Soysal Z, Çakalır C. Forensic Medicine. In: Kolusayın Ö, Koç S, editors. Death. Volume I. İstanbul: İstanbul University Medical Faculty Publications; 1999:93-151

[10] Gök Ş, Tıp A, Ölüm. Filiz Kitabevi. In: Gök Ş, Medicine F, editors. Death. İstanbul: Filiz Publishing House; 1991. pp. 4-34

[11] Maile AE, Inoue CG, Barksdale LE, Carter DO. Toward a universal equation to estimate postmortem interval. Forensic Science International. 2017;**272**:150-153

[12] Shrestha R, Kanchan T, Krishan K. Methods of estimation of time since death. In: StatPearls [Internet]. Treasure Island (FL): StatPearls Publishing; 2023. [Updated 2023 May 30] Available from: https://www.ncbi.nlm.nih.gov/books/NBK549867/

[13] Dix J, Calaluce R. Guide to Forensic Pathology, Time of Death, Decomposition, and Identification. Florida: CRC Press LLC; 1998. pp. 32-48

[14] Di Maio DJ, Di Maio VJM. Forensic Pathology, Time of Death. 2nd ed. Florida: CRC Press LLC; 2001. pp. 43-63

[15] Swift B. The Timing of Death. In: Rutty GN, editor. Essentials of Autopsy Practice. London: Springer; 2006. pp. 189-214. DOI: 10.1007/1-84628-026-5_8

[16] Hirakawa K, Koike K, Uekusa K, Nihira M, Yuta K, Ohno Y. Experimental estimation of postmortem interval using multivariate analysis of proton NMR metabolomic data. Legal Medicine. 2009;**11**(Suppl. 1):S282-S285

[17] Krompecher T, Gilles A, Brandt-Casadevall C, Mangin P. Experimental evaluation of rigor motris IX. The

influence of the breaking (mechanical solution) on the development of rigor motris. Forensic Science International. 2008;**176**:157-162

[18] Shiotani S, Kohno M, Ohashi N, Yamazaki K, Itai Y. Postmortem intravascular high-density fluid level (hypostasis): CT findings. Journal of Computer Assisted Tomography. 2002;**26**(6):892-893

[19] Jackowski C, Thali M, Aghayev E, Yen K, Sonnenschein M, Zwygart K, et al. Postmortem imaging of blood and its characteristics using MSCT and MRI. International Journal of Legal Medicine. 2006;**120**:233-240

[20] Jaafar S, Nokes LDM. Examination of the eye as a means to determine the early postmortem period: A review of the literature. Forensic Science International. 1994;**64**:185-189

[21] Arnaldos MI, García MD, Romera E, Presa JJ, Luna A. Estimation of postmortem interval in real cases based on experimentally obtained entomological evidence. Forensic Science International. 2005;**149**:57-65

[22] Madea B, Musshoff F. Postmortem biochemistry. Forensic Science International. 2007;**165**:165-171

[23] Coe JI. Postmortem chemistry update—Emphasis on forensic applications. The American Journal of Forensic Medicine and Pathology. 1993;**14**(2):91-117

[24] Kominato Y, Kumada K, Yamazaki K, Misawa S. Estimation of postmortem interval based on the third component of complement (C3) cleavage. Journal of Forensic Sciences. 1988;**33**(2):404-409

[25] Endo T, Hara S, Kuriiwa F, Kano S. Postmortem changes in the levels of monoamine metabolites in human cerebrospinal fluid. Forensic Science International. 1990;**44**:61-68

[26] Dogan KH, Günaydin G, Demirci S, Koç S. Postmortem Changes in Element Levels in Rat Skeletal Muscle Tissue/ Siçan Iskelet Kasi Dokusunda Postmortem Element Seviyelerinin Belirlenmesi. Türkiye Klinikleri. Tip Bilimleri Dergisi. 2010;**30**(4):1332

[27] Dell'Aquila M, De Matteis A, Scatena A, Costantino A, Camporeale MC, De Filippis A. Estimation of the time of death: Where we are now? La Clinica Terapeutica. 2021;**172**(2):109-112. DOI: 10.7417/CT.2021.2294

[28] Montanari E, Giorgetti R, Busardò FP, Giorgetti A, Tagliabracci A, Alessandrini F. Suitability of miRNA assessment in postmortem interval estimation. European Review for Medical and Pharmacological Sciences. 2021;**25**(4):1774-1787. DOI: 10.26355/ eurrev_202102_25069

[29] Scrivano S, Sanavio M, Tozzo P, Caenazzo L. Analysis of RNA in the estimation of post-mortem interval: A review of current evidence. International Journal of Legal Medicine. Nov 2019;**133**(6):1629-1640. DOI: 10.1007/ s00414-019-02125-x

[30] Peng D, Lv M, Li Z, Tian H, Qu S, Jin B, et al. Postmortem interval determination using mRNA markers and DNA normalization. International Journal of Legal Medicine. Jan 2020;**134**(1):149-157. DOI: 10.1007/s00414-019-02199-7

[31] Sangwan A, Singh SP, Singh P, Gupta OP, Manas A. Gupta S, role of molecular techniques in PMI estimation: An update. Journal of Forensic and Legal Medicine. 2021;**83**:102251. DOI: 10.1016/j.jflm.2021.102251. ISSN 1752-928X

Chapter 7

Histopathological Changes in Liver in Autopsies

Shivani Gandhi, Reetika Menia, Ishani Gupta and Surbhi Mahajan

Abstract

Histopathological examination is one of the important ancillary investigations to be done in medicolegal autopsies, particularly in sudden and natural deaths. Some of the liver diseases are silent that can contribute to fatal events in the later stages. Liver is one of the common viscera received in the pathology laboratory for histopathological examination. The findings in the liver vary from nonspecific to specific, which may or may not contribute to the cause of death. The important prerequisite for the histopathological examination is preservation. A well-preserved specimen gives detailed morphological details when compared to the poorly preserved specimen.

Keywords: liver, histopathology, post-mortem, examination, hepatic

1. Introduction

The liver is vulnerable to a number of injuries, which may be metabolic, microbial, toxic, or traumatic. Although liver is known for its vast regenerative capacity, many serious injuries cause permanent damage, which is beyond its regenerative ability. Most hepatic injuries can be diagnosed on histopathology using liver biopsy but many fatal conditions remain undiagnosed and are studied at autopsy. Hepatic injuries may be acute or chronic. The disease condition lasting more than six months is labeled as chronic [1]. Thus, liver autopsy serves as an eminent tool in helping pathologists reach a definitive diagnosis and forensic experts to specify the cause of death and to plan medical intervention [2]. Gross and microscopic examination of the autopsy specimen of liver gives clues about the underlying diseased conditions. Abnormal liver biopsies on histopathology often reveal—liver cirrhosis, infarcts, fatty change, glycogen storage disease, tuberculosis, acute poisoning, hemosiderosis, hyperemia, amyloidosis, abscess, syphilis, actinomycosis, hydatid cyst, and malignancy [3]. Alcohol abuse is one of the major causes of pathological liver diseases such as fatty liver, alcoholic cirrhosis, and hepatitis. These disease conditions may all be seen concomitantly in one patient [4].

Abnormal findings in liver autopsy can be fatty change, hepar lobatum, glycogen storage disease, acute phosphorus poisoning, hemosiderosis, syphilis, actinomycosis, infarcts, cloudy swelling, tuberculosis, acute passive hyperemia, chronic passive hyperemia, amyloidosis, abscess, hydatid cyst, malignancy, cirrhosis, and acute yellow atrophy [3].

Autopsy is usually performed in cases of road trauma accidents, railway accidents, burns, drowning, poisoning, tuberculosis, etc. A careful autopsy examination both gross and microscopic is required to study in depth the disease etiology and the site of origin to differentiate between primary and secondary liver diseases and to reach a definitive diagnosis. After conducting the gross study, the sections taken for microscopy are stained with hematoxylin and eosin (H&E), evaluated and then, appropriate special stains are applied, as the need may arise.

The morphological findings of the liver or part of a liver received after the post-mortem in the Department of Pathology are discussed in detail as under:

2. Hepatic cirrhosis

Hepatic cirrhosis is diagnosed on histopathology. The histopathological findings include the loss of normal architecture with loss of normal central-portal relationships [5]. The specimen examined must be large with several intact portal and central areas. Grossly and microscopically, it is characterized by the formation of nodules, as depicted in **Figures 1–3**.

There are three main forms of hepatic cirrhosis according to the pathomorphological classification which classifies cirrhosis based on the diameter of the connective tissue nodes:

a. Micronodular form of hepatic cirrhosis (MNHC), where the diameter of connective tissue nodes is less than 3 millimeters (nodule size in the range of 1–3 mm);

b. Coarse nodular form of hepatic cirrhosis (CNHC) where the diameter of nodules is more than 3 mm; and

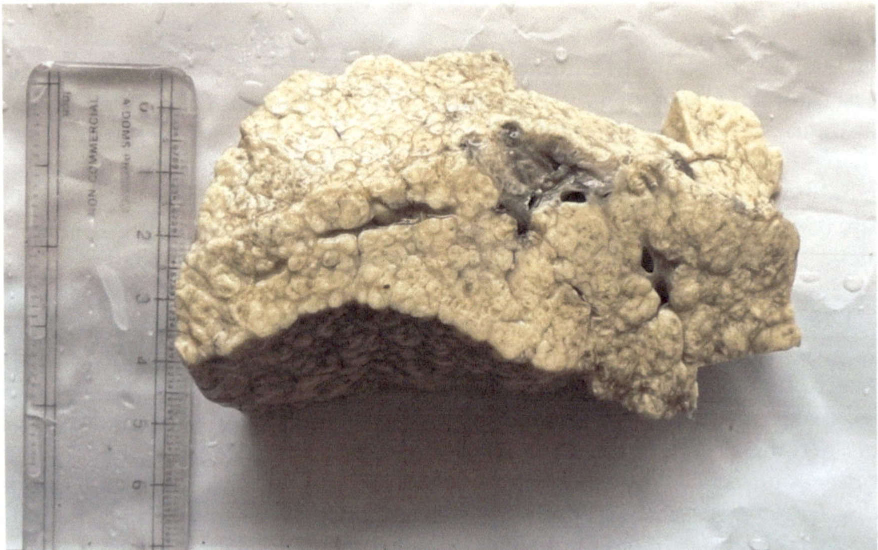

Figure 1.
Mixed nodular cirrhosis of liver at autopsy. Cut section of the liver shows nodular appearance, size of each nodule varying from 1 mm to 10 mm. The normal architecture of the liver parenchyma has been distorted by these nodular formations.

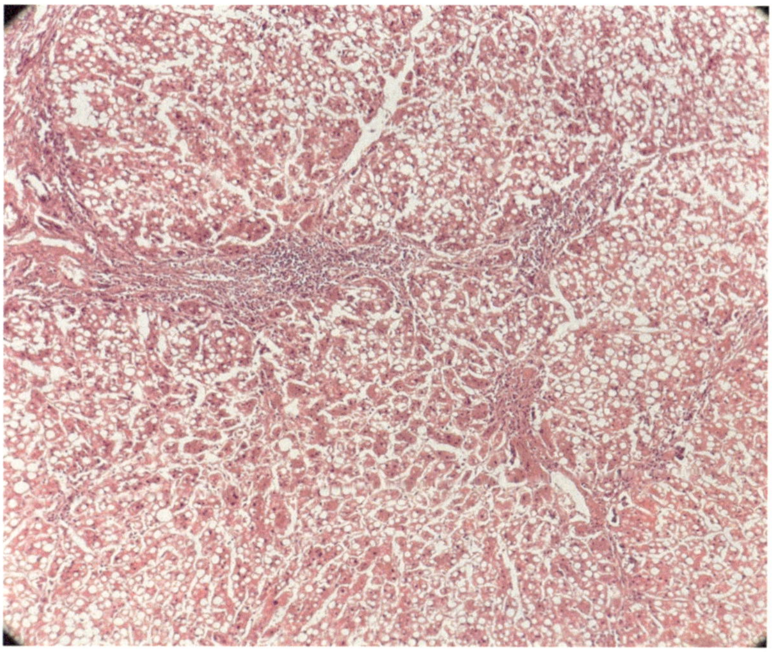

Figure 2.
Micropictograph of a section of a liver depicting the cirrhosis characterized by loss of architecture and presence of regenerating nodules separated by bands of fibrosis (hematoxylin and eosin (H&E), 40×).

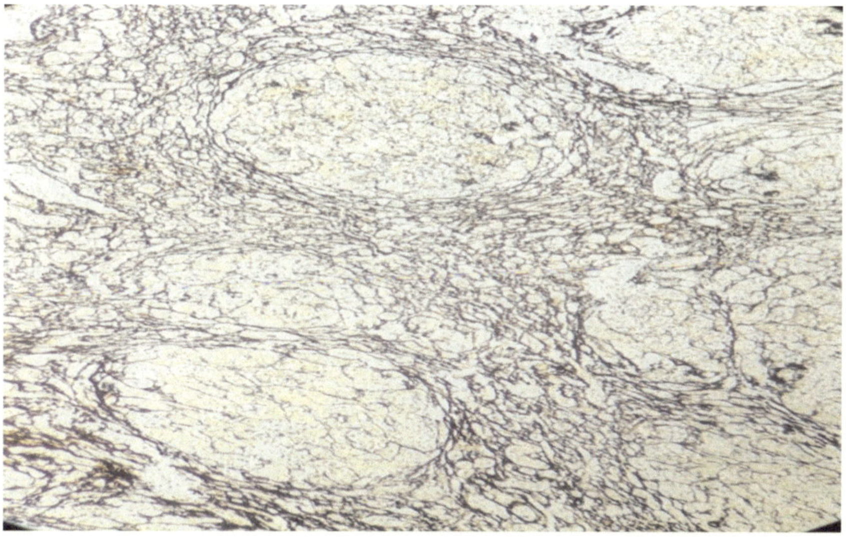

Figure 3.
The reticulin stain for reticular fibers depicting the connective tissue septa surrounding the regenerating nodules and the general increase in connective tissue fibers (fibrosis) (hematoxylin and eosin (H&E), 40×).

c. Mixed hepatic cirrhosis (MHC), which involves both small and large nodules in the liver parenchyma [3].

Morphological changes taking into consideration the severity of destructive and dystrophic changes in structure are used to classify the stage of liver failure. As per this concept, all deaths by hepatic cirrhosis can be divided into three groups, each of which corresponded to a certain stage of liver failure as follows:

i. Compensated stage of liver failure (CSLF) with initial morphological changes, where changes are seen only in the hepatoportal sections of the hepatic acini.

ii. Decompensated stage of liver failure (DSLF) or a stage of pronounced changes, when destructive and dystrophic changes are detected throughout both the hepatoportal sections and hepatic tubules of the hepatic acini.

iii. The end-stage of liver failure (ESLF), when during histological examination changes are seen in all three sections of the hepatic acini: hepatoportal, tubular, and the central vein area.

3. Hepatitis

It can be acute or chronic. In acute hepatitis, there may be focal/multifocal necrosis that does not follow a zonal pattern but involves random, individual clusters of hepatocytes. Acute hepatitis also includes ballooning degeneration of hepatocytes, lobular and sinusoidal inflammation, Kupffer cell hyperplasia, increased apoptotic bodies, and cholestasis. If this process lasts longer than six months, it is deemed chronic and often presents progressive fibrosis [6].

3.1 Chronic hepatitis

It is defined as a liver disease with persistent necro-inflammatory activity lasting more than six months. The most common causes of chronic hepatitis are viral, auto-immune, and drug-induced.

3.1.1 Gross findings

Liver may appear grossly normal in the early stages of chronic hepatitis. In later stages, the hepatic parenchyma is firm because of increased fibrosis. Cirrhosis due to viral hepatitis is generally macronodular.

3.1.2 Microscopic findings

In chronic hepatitis, there is focal necrosis of hepatocytes at the limiting plate between the portal tract connective tissue and the beginning of hepatic parenchyma with an associated lymphocytic infiltrate—called piecemeal necrosis or interface hepatitis, necrosis and fibrosis are seen in later stages.

In most cases of chronic hepatitis, there is portal inflammation characterized by the presence of a prominent inflammatory infiltrate consisting of lymphocytes with a variable number of plasma cells involving the portal tracts. Scattered macrophages, neutrophils, and eosinophils are typically a minor component of the infiltrate. Lymphoid follicles and germinal centers may be seen. Bile duct reaction may be seen at the periphery of the portal tract. Interface hepatitis, also known as piecemeal necrosis or periportal necrosis, is an important feature of chronic hepatitis. The lymphocytes and plasma cells of the inflammatory periportal infiltrate are closely associated with degenerating hepatocytes at the limiting plate. Hepatocytes, in areas of piecemeal necrosis, often undergo ballooning degeneration and appear pale and swollen with clumping of cytoplasm. Apoptotic bodies may also be seen in areas of active interface hepatitis. The periportal parenchyma is gradually destroyed and replaced by fibrosis. Hepatocyte necrosis in chronic hepatitis is variable in severity but usually spotty. Apoptotic hepatocytes (acidophil bodies) are scattered throughout the lobule. Mononuclear inflammatory cells cluster around injured hepatocytes and may obscure focal hepatocyte necrosis. Kupffer cells in these areas of spotty hepatocyte necrosis may contain phagocytosed cellular debris. Ballooning degeneration may be seen in the exacerbation of chronic viral hepatitis and may be associated with zone 3 cholestasis. Regeneration of hepatocytes is recognizable by the formation of liver cell plates that are two cells thick and by the formation of regenerating rosettes.

3.1.3 Fibrosis

Progressive fibrosis at the limiting plate as the result of continued necro-inflammatory activity leads to stellate enlargement of the portal tract. Portal-portal fibrous septa are the result of the linkage of adjacent fibrotic portal tracts. Portal central fibrous bridging can also develop generally from superimposed episodes of severe lobular necro-inflammatory activity involving zone 3. The end result of bridging fibrosis is cirrhosis, which is usually macronodular or mixed micro- and macronodular. Other hepatocyte changes seen in chronic hepatitis include steatosis, iron deposition, and oncocyte change. The scoring system based on the inflammation and lobular activity is used for grading chronic hepatitis, whereas staging depends upon the fibrosis as depicted in **Table 1**.

Grade	
A. Portal inflammation and interface hepatitis	
0	Absent or minimal
1	Portal inflammation only
2	Mild or localized interface hepatitis
3	Moderate or more extensive interface hepatitis
4	Severe and widespread interface hepatitis
B. Lobular activity	
0	None
1	Inflammatory cells but no hepatocellular damage
2	Focal necrosis or apoptosis
3	Severe hepatocellular damage
4	Damage includes bridging confluent necrosis
Stage	
0	No fibrosis
1	Fibrosis confined to portal tracts
2	Periportal or portal-portal septa but intact vascular relationships
3	Fibrosis with distorted structure but no obvious cirrhosis
4	Probable or definite cirrhosis

Table 1.
A simple scoring system for chronic hepatitis.

4. Chronic venous congestion

The hepatic manifestations due to circulatory compromise lead to venous congestion. Chronic venous congestion and centrilobular necrosis are commonly seen at autopsy because there is an element of preterminal circulatory failure with virtually every death [7]. Right-sided cardiac decompensation leads to passive congestion of the liver. The liver is slightly enlarged, tense, and cyanotic with round edges. The liver takes on a variegated mottled appearance, known traditionally as the 'Nutmeg' Liver. Microscopically, there is congestion of centrilobular sinusoids (**Figure 4**) [8]. Left-sided cardiac failure or shock may lead to hepatic hypoperfusion and hypoxia. The hepatocytes in the central region of the lobule undergo ischemic necrosis and centrilobular necrosis is visible microscopically as a slight depression of necrotic lobular centers. By microscopy, there is a sharp demarcation of viable hepatocytes in the periportal region versus necrotic hepatocytes in the centrilobular region of the parenchyma. Congestion alone, no matter how severe or prolonged, seems to do little if any damage to the liver. Centrilobular necrosis or ischemic hepatitis appears to result from hepatic hypoperfusion and mimics viral hepatitis [7].

5. Granulomatous lesions of liver

Granulomatous lesions of liver are seen in 2–10% liver biopsies [9]. These are seen in various systemic conditions or may be noticed as incidental findings in an otherwise normal liver biopsy. The structural liver damage is rarely caused by the granulomas themselves, but their detection can be the first indication of an underlying systemic disease.

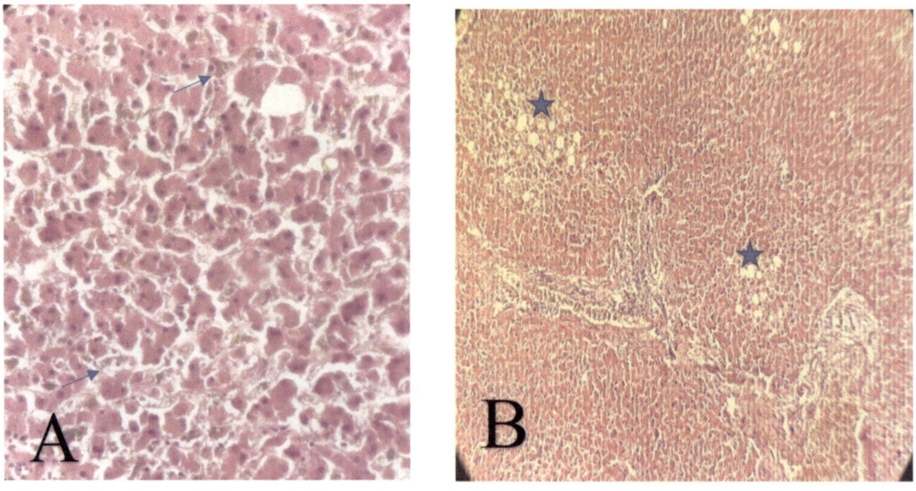

Figure 4.
Light micrograph of a section through the liver with chronic venous congestion depicting red blood cells (RBCs) are phagocytosed by macrophages, which are called siderophages (depicted with arrows in A) and central vein and sinusoids are distended with RBCs along with the presence of fatty change (depicted with star in B).

5.1 Causes of hepatic granuloma

Granulomatous lesions of liver are associated with various disorders (**Table 2**). In the West, most common causes are sarcoidosis, drug-induced, tuberculosis, neoplastic disease, and primary biliary cholangitis [10].

5.2 Histopathology

Granulomas are well-circumscribed lesions that are formed as a result of an inflammatory reaction. They have a central core of macrophages, with a surrounding

Causes of granulomatous lesions in liver		
Autoimmune diseases	Sarcoidosis Primary biliary cirrhosis	
Infections	Bacterial	Tuberculosis Brucellosis Secondary syphilis Listeriosis *Mycobacterium avium* complex Lepromatous leprosy Cat scratch fever Leishmaniasis
	Viral	Cytomegalovirus Hepatitis A, B, and C Epstein-Barr virus
	Fungal	Histoplasmosis Cryptococcus Candidiasis Nocardiosis Coccidioidomycosis
	Parasitic	Schistosomiasis Toxoplasmosis
Vasculitides	Polyarteritis nodosa Churg-Strauss syndrome Granulomatosis with polyangiitis	
Drugs	Nitrofurantoin Allopurinol Phenytoin	
Malignancy	Hodgkin's lymphoma and non-Hodgkin's lymphoma Renal cell carcinoma Hepatic metastases	
Inherited	Chronic granulomatous diseases	
Ingestion of foreign body	Mineral oil, talc, or starch	
Metal toxicity	Copper toxicity Berylliosis	
Chronic gastrointestinal disease	Crohn's disease	
Idiopathic		

Table 2.
Causes of granulomatous lesions in liver.

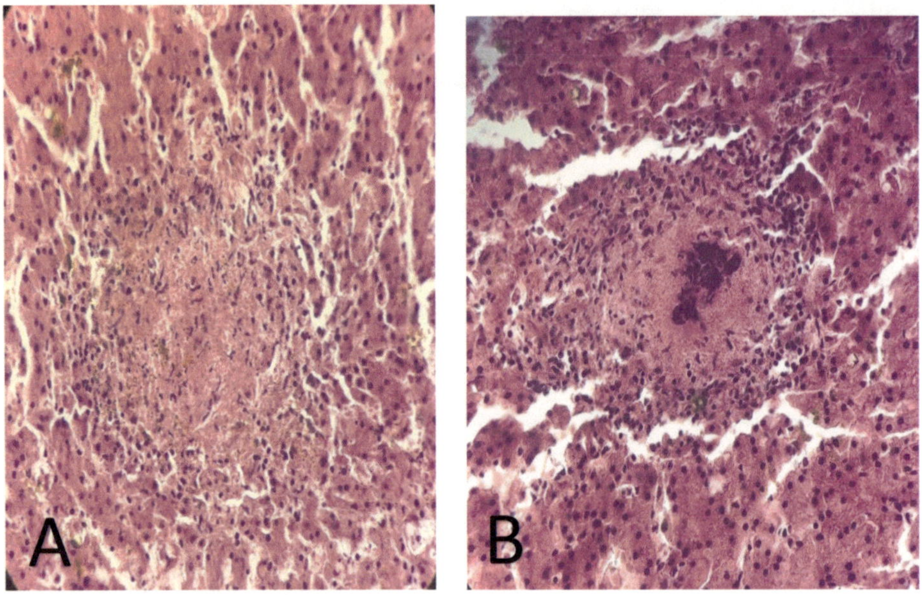

Figure 5.
Photomicrograph of liver biopsy from a patient at autopsy showing epithelioid cell (A) and giant cell granulomas (B) (hematoxylin and eosin (H&E), 40×).

Histological variants of hepatic granulomas			
S. no.	**Variant**	**Histological feature**	**Causes**
1.	Noncaseating	They do not have necrosis	Sarcoidosis
2.	Caseating	They have central core of caseous necrosis	Tuberculosis Granulomatosis with polyangitis
3.	Fibrin-ring	The epithelioid cells surround a vacuole within an encircling fibrin ring	Hodgkin's lymphoma, Leishmaniasis, Q fever, giant cell arteritis, allopurinol
4.	Lipogranulomas	These granulomas contain a central lipid vacuole	Ingestion of mineral oil, hepatic steatosis

Table 3.
The different histological variants of hepatic granulomas.

rim that consists of lymphocytes, plasma cells, giant cells, and fibroblasts, as depicted in **Figure 5**. There are four main histological types of hepatic granulomas, which are described in **Table 3**.

The granulomas are mostly located in the hepatic parenchyma but in certain conditions like primary biliary cholangitis, they are located in the portal tracts.

Special stains like acid-fast and fungal staining can be used for visualization of the concerned microorganisms in the liver biopsy, which can aid in reaching the diagnosis.

6. Liver abscess

Liver abscess is a pus-filled cavity in the liver which can develop due to any injury to the liver or any intra-abdominal infection which is disseminated through the portal circulation [11]. They can be categorized into pyogenic or amoebic, although a few of them can also be caused by parasites and fungi. *Entamoeba histolytica* is the main offending agent observed in amoebic liver abscess. *Pyogenic* abscess is most commonly caused by *Escherichia coli* (*E.coli*), *Klebsiella*, *Streptococcus*, *Staphylococcus*, and anaerobes.

Around 40–50 million people are annually infected with amoebic abscesses and the majority of infections occur in developing countries [12, 13]. The prevalence of infection in endemic areas is higher than 10% and in certain areas, it is reported to be as high as 55%. Amoebic liver abscesses are the most common extraintestinal manifestation of *Entamoeba histolytica* infection. The incidence of Pyogenic liver abscess in the USA is 2.3 per 1,00,000 [14]. *Streptococcus milleri* is the most common pathogen followed by *Klebsiella pneumoniae* found in Pyogenic liver abscess.

The abscess is formed mostly due to leakage from the bowel in the abdomen, which travels through the portal vein to the liver. Biliary tract infection, which has direct contact with liver, can also cause abscess.

The classification of liver abscesses can be done by various methods: One of the methods is by its location in the liver. Liver abscess is seen more commonly in the right lobe of the liver because of its blood supply as compared to the left liver lobe or caudate lobe. Another method is the cause of liver abscess. If it is infectious, then most of them can be classified into bacterial (amoebic) and parasitic (hydatiform cyst).

6.1 Pathogenesis

Pyogenic abscess is defined as a collection of pus which consists of many inflammatory cells, mainly neutrophils and tissue debris [15]. Necrosis is also associated with the infection. In amoebic liver abscess, hepatocyte cell death occurs either by apoptosis or by necrosis [16]. The inflammatory cells are absent due to the lysis of neutrophils by the protozoan, thus forming the nonpurulent 'anchovy paste' abscess [17]. Expansion of the abscess with cell death continues until the treatment of the patient starts.

7. Steatohepatitis

Nonalcoholic fatty liver disease (NAFLD) is one of the most common liver diseases in developed countries. It is defined as the accumulation of fat within liver cells in individuals who do not have a history of alcohol ingestion [18]. Nonalcoholic fatty liver disease (NAFLD) and nonalcoholic steatohepatitis (NASH) are diagnosed on the basis of histological findings of either fat alone, fat along with inflammation, fat with ballooning degeneration, or fat along with fibrosis and cirrhosis [19]. The prevalence and clinical outcome of these vary according to the histological category [20].

Nonalcoholic fatty liver disease (NAFLD) is commonly noted in obese individuals. Around 74–90% of liver biopsies of such individuals show fatty change [21]. Ludwig et al. coined the term NASH [22]. It is less aggressive as compared to alcoholic hepatitis but can progress through necro-inflammatory change and early fibrosis to cirrhosis [23].

8. Fatty liver

One of the common findings seen in the liver both in the autopsy and clinical settings is fatty liver or steatosis. It is frequently associated with alcohol abuse and also seen in nonalcoholic fatty liver disease (NAFLD), resulting in end-stage hepatic failure. Abnormal retention of fat vacuoles or triglycerides in hepatocytes leads to fatty change, which in turn constitutes liver disease. Nonalcoholic fatty liver disease (NAFLD) is characterized by excessive fat accumulation in hepatic parenchyma ($\geq$ 5%) in the absence of excessive alcohol intake (< 20 g/day). As per the World Health Organization (WHO), mortality related to alcohol consumption is 3.8% globally and the prevalence of nonalcoholic steatohepatitis in India ranges from 5 to 28% [24]. It is one of the frequent findings at autopsy, seen in all age groups [25]. The main etiological factors that constitute chronic liver disease worldwide are chronic alcohol abuse followed by virus-induced hepatitis and NAFLD [26]. The prevalence of fatty liver among the population depends upon the technique being used for the diagnosis, which can range from imaging to biopsy, each having different accuracy levels in different settings. It is considered a marker of other disorders that can be one of the causes of death. The twelfth leading cause of death in the USA is attributed to chronic liver diseases and cirrhosis, with NAFLD being rapidly increasing in the USA as well as in other developed worlds within this subcategory [27].

Steatosis is one of the most common findings seen microscopically and it can be microvesicular or macrovesicular, the latter being more common. Macrovesicular steatosis is characterized by the presence of a single fat vacuole in the hepatocyte that displaces the nucleus toward the edge, whereas in microvesicular steatosis, there are multiple small vacuoles in the cytoplasm with a centrally placed nucleus. The histological findings in fatty liver include the presence of steatosis that can range from mild to more severe forms along with lobular and/or portal inflammation, hepatocyte ballooning, and fibrosis that may vary in distribution, as shown in **Figures 6** and 7.

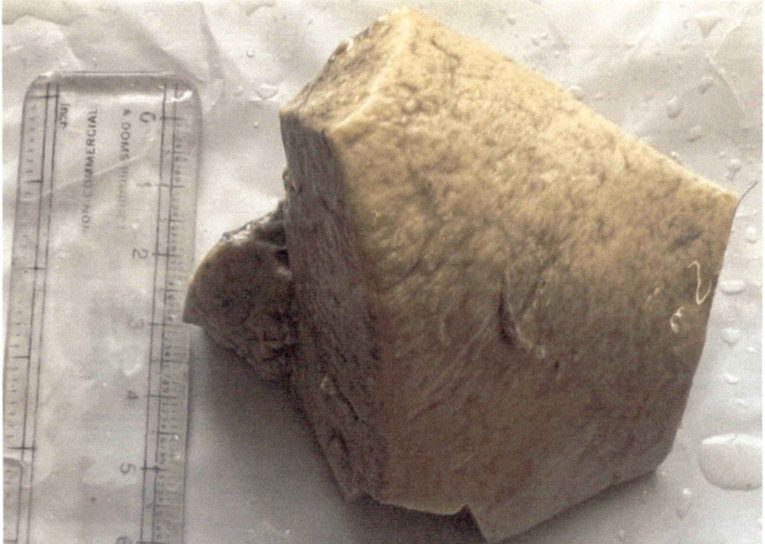

Figure 6.
Gross photograph of the liver tissue illustrates the yellowish color of the liver parenchyma. The yellow color indicates high fat content in this tissue.

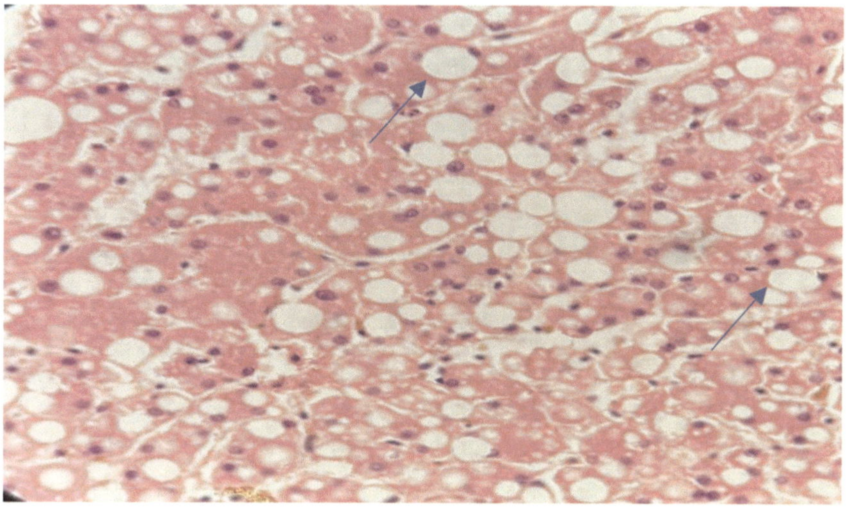

Figure 7.
Micropictograph of fatty change in hepatocytes with lipid vacuoles. In many cells, the nucleus is displaced to the periphery of the cell and the entire cytoplasm is taken up by the giant lipid vacuole (shown with arrow). (hematoxylin and eosin (H&E), 40×).

9. Structural abnormalities

Many chronic liver diseases may remain silent and may undergo undiagnosed during their lifetime. These diseases may be found as incidental findings during routine body checkup or investigations for other diseases or at autopsy. Liver abnormalities can be structural, congenital, or vascular or abnormalities of the bile duct [28].

The major congenital abnormalities of liver are listed in **Table 4**.

(A) Structural abnormalities of liver		
S. no	**Abnormality**	**Features**
a.	Agenesis/absence of liver	Autopsy finding in stillbirths
b.	Agenesis of lobe of liver	
c.	Hypoplasia of right lobe	Is a rare condition, can be seen associated with suprahepatic or retrohepatic gallbladder
d.	*Situs inversus totalis* or *abdominalis*	*Characterized by abnormal position of the liver in left hypochondrium*
e.	*Riedel lobe*	*Accessory hepatic lobe seen as a tongue-like projection from the right lobe*
f.	*Ectopic hepatic tissue*	*Found in* suspensory ligaments of the liver, lung, wall of the gallbladder, splenic capsule, greater omentum, etc.
(B) Vascular anomalies that can involve portal vein or hepatic artery are:		
a.	Preduodenal portal vein	Can result in duodenal obstruction, causing gastric outlet obstruction in adults
b.	Aberrant hepatic arteries	Can be present in association with biliary atresia

(B) Vascular anomalies that can involve portal vein or hepatic artery are:

S. No	Abnormality	Features
c.	Presence of obstructing valves within splenic vein or portal vein	Is a rare cause of portal hypertension in children
d.	Duplication of portal vein	
e.	Atresia/hypoplasia of portal vein	It may involve the entire length or part of a vessel
f.	Congenital absence of portal vein	Is a rare entity in children, with a few cases also having been reported in adults
g.	Portal cavernoma	Also known as cavernous transformation of portal vein characterized by the replacement of vein by trabeculated venous lake that are spongy and extend to gastroduodenal ligament
h.	Congenital shunts	Can be portohepatic, portocaval, or between left portal vein and internal mammary veins

(C) Anomalies involving bile duct are listed

S. No	Abnormality	Features
a.	Agenesis of the common bile duct	*Is a rare entity*
b.	Agenesis of the common hepatic duct	*Obstructive jaundice is a common presenting complaint*
c.	Anomalous insertion of the right hepatic duct	*Is also a rare entity*
d.	Anomalous ('accessory') bile ducts	
e.	Duplication of the bile ducts	One duct may empty into the pylorus or both may drain into the duodenum
f.	Ciliated hepatic foregut cyst	Is a rare entity, more common in men, involving the medial segment of the left hepatic lobe.

Table 4.
The major congenital abnormalities of liver.

10. Nodules

Nodules in the liver can be found as an incidental finding at autopsy. These nodules may vary in size and may occur singly or as multiple lesions. The nodular lesions in liver may be benign or malignant. The differential diagnosis of benign nodules includes hepatic hemangioma, hepatocellular adenoma, regenerative nodules, hepatic cyst, focal nodular hyperplasia, liver abscess, compensatory hyperplasia, focal fatty change, whereas the malignant lesions include hepatocellular carcinoma, dysplastic nodules, cholangiocarcinoma, liver metastasis, and rarely lymphoma.

11. Alcoholic liver disease and nonalcoholic fatty liver disease

Alcohol-associated liver disease (ALD) and nonalcoholic fatty liver disease (NAFLD) are significant global health issues. These two conditions share similar pathological characteristics, encompassing a spectrum from simple hepatic steatosis to steatohepatitis, liver cirrhosis, and hepatocellular carcinoma [29]. Alcohol-associated liver disease (ALD) alone accounts for 5.1% of all worldwide disease and injury burdens, often resulting in earlier mortality and disability compared to other chronic liver injuries [30]. Nonalcoholic fatty liver disease (NAFLD) is diagnosed clinically and is characterized by the presence of 5% or more hepatic steatosis, as determined by liver imaging or biopsy, in the absence of secondary causes of hepatic fat accumulation (such as alcohol, hepatitis C virus (HCV), Wilson's disease, medications, etc.). It is a metabolic disorder influenced by hormonal, nutritional, and genetic factors [31].

Gross features of ALD:

- Early stage: enlarged, soft, greasy, yellow liver
- Late stage: shrunken, mottled, red-brown liver with bile staining
- End-stage: cirrhosis

Histopathological findings:

- Steatosis (accumulation of fat)
- Zone 3 injury pattern
- Ballooning degeneration
- Lobular inflammatory infiltrates, particularly rich in neutrophils
- Mallory hyaline
- Perivenular fibrosis
- Pericellular fibrosis
- Bile ductular reaction [32]

The fatty degeneration of liver cells occurs to a greater degree in NAFLD than in ALD. In contrast, inflammatory cell infiltration is more pronounced in ALD than in NAFLD. Furthermore, venous or perivenular fibrosis, phlebosclerosis, and (less commonly) lymphocytic phlebitis are more common in ALD than in NAFLD [29].

12. Leukemic infiltrates

Hematopoietic tumors of the liver are infrequently encountered by practicing pathologists due to the rarity of primary hepatic lesions and the fact that many cases of leukemia and lymphoma involving the liver are not biopsied [33]. While hepatic involvement in acute leukemia is typically mild and asymptomatic during diagnosis, a post-mortem study revealed liver infiltration in over 95% of acute lymphoblastic leukemia (ALL) cases and up to 75% of acute myeloid leukemia (AML) cases. Massive infiltration of leukemic cells in the liver can manifest as fulminant hepatic failure [34].

In almost all cases, myeloid tumors of the liver indicate hepatic involvement by myeloid leukemias, although rare instances of hepatic myeloid sarcomas have been reported. In the chronic phase, approximately 50% of chronic myeloid leukemia (CML) patients show mild to moderate hepatomegaly at presentation, without liver function abnormalities. However, during blastic crisis, sinusoidal infiltration of immature cells may lead to liver enlargement and elevated serum alkaline phosphatase (ALP) levels.

Primary hepatic lymphoma is a rare form of liver malignancy. The most common subtype is diffuse large B-cell lymphoma, a type of non-Hodgkin's lymphoma that frequently occurs outside of lymph nodes. Hepatic involvement with lymphoma cells and hepatomegaly is more common in non-Hodgkin's lymphoma (NHL) compared to Hodgkin's lymphoma (HL), with 16–43% of NHL cases showing liver involvement. Extrahepatic obstruction is also more prevalent in NHL compared to HL. Liver infiltration by malignant cells has been reported in 14% of HL patients. Hepatomegaly is found in 9% of patients with stage I-II disease and in 45% of patients with stage III-I disease [34].

Another rare subtype is hepatosplenic T-cell lymphoma, which primarily affects young adult males.

Patterns of hepatic involvement in important leukemic infiltrates include:

- Acute myeloid leukemia-Sinusoids, portal tracts, and even individual hepatocytes. If the infiltrate forms a distinct mass that disrupts the hepatic architecture, it is termed a myeloid sarcoma.
- Acute lymphoblastic leukemia-Portal tracts.
- Chronic myelogenous leukemia-Distension of hepatic sinusoids by neoplastic cells, although variable-sized infiltrates in the portal tracts can also be present.
- Hepatosplenic T-cell lymphoma is characterized by sinusoidal infiltration by uniform medium-sized lymphocytes [33].

13. Metastasis

The liver is a common site for cancer metastasis, accounting for approximately 25% of all cases. Metastatic carcinomas are more frequently encountered than primary liver tumors. The presence of hepatic metastases increases the morbidity and mortality of patients with primary tumors in other sites, including the colon, breast, pancreas, lung, kidney, and stomach. The dual blood supply of the liver makes it susceptible to metastasis from gastrointestinal cancers and allows for interventional therapies. However, metastases are relatively uncommon in cirrhotic livers [35].

They typically appear as discrete and well-demarcated lesions, both grossly and histologically, separate from the surrounding liver tissue often with a hyperemic rim and can be single or multiple. In some cases, they may display infiltrative growth, resembling intrahepatic cholangiocarcinoma or hepatocellular carcinoma (HCC). Diffuse infiltrative patterns can also resemble primary liver tumors [32].

14. Carcinoma

Hepatocellular carcinoma (HCC) is the primary tumor that originates in the liver and accounts for over 90% of all primary liver tumors. It is currently the fifth most common cancer worldwide. Among men, HCC is the second leading cause of cancer-related deaths following lung cancer. The major risk factors for hepatocellular carcinoma include viral hepatitis (hepatitis B and hepatitis C), alcoholic liver disease, and nonalcoholic fatty liver disease (NAFLD) or steatohepatitis [36].

Gross pathology:

- Nodules that are soft, yellow-green, or reddish in color
- Variable sizes, ranging from small to large
- Different types, including solitary, multinodular, and diffuse

Histopathology:
Three classic patterns: trabecular, acinar, and solid

- Trabecular pattern: thick cords lined by flat endothelial cells, lacking Kupffer cells
- Acinar pattern: central degeneration of solid trabeculae, leading to pseudoglandular spaces containing colloid-like material or bile; may also involve dilated canaliculi
- Solid pattern: resulting from compression artifacts or scarring; the least common of the three patterns

The cytological features of HCC depend on the level of hepatocyte differentiation, ranging from well differentiated to poorly differentiated.

15. Conclusion

The liver is a common site for various diseases, of which many are symptomatic, whereas others may remain silent or asymptomatic and a few are found only at autopsy. Having a vast reserve, many liver diseases remain silent most of the time. Thus, the histopathological study of liver specimens at post-mortem examination is an important learning modality for both pathologists and clinicians to study silent liver diseases, to further improve the clinical and diagnostic approach toward diseases of the liver.

Author details

Shivani Gandhi[1*], Reetika Menia[1], Ishani Gupta[1] and Surbhi Mahajan[2]

1 Department of Pathology, All India Institute of Medical Sciences, Jammu, J&K, India

2 Department of Pathology, Government Medical College, Jammu, J&K, India

*Address all correspondence to: dr.shivanigandhi@gmail.com

References

[1] Butler DC, Lewin DN, Batalis NI. Differential diagnosis of hepatic necrosis encountered at autopsy. Academic Forensic Pathology. 2018;**8**(2):256-295

[2] Umesh BR, Gayathri BN, Harendra Kumar ML. Spectrum of liver pathology at autopsy. International Journal of Research and Review. 2015;**2**(3):79-86

[3] Sotoudehmanesh R, Sotoudeh M, Ali-Asgari A, Abedi-Ardakani B, Tavangar SM, Khakinejad A, et al. Silent liver diseases in autopsies from forensic medicine of Tehran. Archives of Iranian Medicine. 2006;**9**(4):324-328

[4] Subedi N, Yadav BN, Jha S, Gurung S, Pradhan A. An autopsy study of liver injuries in a Tertiary Referral Centre of eastern Nepal. Journal of Clinical and Diagnostic Research. 2013;**7**(8): 1686-1688

[5] Noritake K, Unuma K, Nara A, Uchida K, Shiratori T, Watanuki Y, et al. Autopsy findings of a patient with rapidly progressive massive ascites caused by alcoholic cirrhosis. Legal Medicine (Tokyo, Japan). 2011;**13**(3): 148-150

[6] Pigolkin YI, Morozov YE, Globa IV, Nikolenko VN. Hepatic cirrhosis according to the forensic medical autopsy data from Moscow for the period of 2007–2016. Russian Open Medical Journal. 2019;**8**:e0412

[7] Chu CW, Hwang SJ, Luo JC, et al. Comparison of clinical, virologic and pathologic features in patients with acute hepatitis B&C. Journal of Gastroenterology and Hepatology. 2001; **16**:209-214

[8] Monte SM, Arcidi JM, Moore GW, Hutchins GM. Midzonal necrosis of hepatocellular injury after shock. Gastroentrology. 1984;**86**:627

[9] Lamps L. Hepatic granulomas: A review with an emphasis on infectious causes. Archives of Pathology & Laboratory Medicine. 2015;**139**:867-875

[10] Lagana SM, Moreira RK, Lefkowitch JH. Hepatic granulomas: Pathogenesis and differential diagnosis. Clinics in Liver Disease. 2010;**14**:605-617

[11] Mischnik A, Kern WV, Thimme R. Pyogenic liver abscess: Changes of organisms and consequences for diagnosis and therapy. Deutsche Medizinische Wochenschrift. 2017 Jul; **142**(14):1067-1074

[12] Bhatti A, Ali F, Satti S, Satti T. Clinical & pathological comparison of pyogenic and amoebic liver abscess. Advances in Infectious Diseases. 2014;**4**: 77-123

[13] Brandt H, Tamayo RP. Pathology of human Amebiasis. Human Pathology. 1970;**1**(3):351-381

[14] Kaplan GG, Gregson DB, Laupland KB. Population based study of the epidemiology of and the risk factors for pyogenic liver abscess. Clinical Gastroenterology and Hepatology. 2004; **2**:1032-1038

[15] De Souza Andrade-Filho J. Revista do Instituto de Medicina Tropical de São Paulo. 2012. Available from: http://www.scielo.br/scielo.php?script=sci_arttext&pid=S0036-46652012000400011

[16] Prakash V, Oliver TI. In: Abai B, Abu-Ghosh A, Acharya AB, et al., editors. Amoebic Liver Abscess. Florida: StatPearls Publishing; 2019 Available

from: https://www.ncbi.nlm.nih.gov/books/NBK430832/

[17] Sifri CD, Madoff LC. Infections of the liver and biliary system (liver abscess, cholangitis, cholecystitis). In: Bennett JE, Dolin R, Blaser MJ, editors. Principles and Practice of Infectious Diseases. 8th ed. Philadelphia: Elsevier Saunders; 2015. pp. 1270-1279

[18] Ong JP, Younossi ZM. Epidemiology and natural history of NAFLD and NASH. Clinics in Liver Disease. 2007;**11**:1-16 vii

[19] Angulo P. Nonalcoholic fatty liver disease. The New England Journal of Medicine. 2002;**346**:1221-1231

[20] Youssef WI, McCullough AJ. Steatohepatitis in obese individuals. Best Practice & Research Clinical Gastroenterology. 2002;**16**:733-747

[21] Luyckx FH, Desaive C, Thiry A, Dewé W, Scheen AJ, Gielen JE, et al. Liver abnormalities in severely obese subjects: Effect of drastic weight loss after gastroplasty. International Journal of Obesity and Related Metabolic Disorders. 1998;**22**:222-226

[22] Ludwig J, Viggiano TR, McGill DB, Oh BJ. Nonalcoholic steatohepatitis: Mayo Clinic experiences with a hitherto unnamed disease. Mayo Clinic Proceedings. 1980;**55**:434-438

[23] Sheth SG, Gordon FD, Chopra S. Nonalcoholic steatohepatitis. Annals of Internal Medicine. 1997;**126**:137-145

[24] Porwal V, Mishra N, Jain D, Gupta S. Post mortem study of alcoholic and non-alcoholic liver diseases in Ajmer region. Annals of Pathology and Laboratory Medicine. 2020;7(5):229-235

[25] Milroy CM. Fatty liver and the forensic pathologist. Academic Forensic Pathology. 2018;**8**(2):296-310. DOI: 10.1177/1925362118782061

[26] Mokdad AA, Lopez AD, Shahraz S, et al. Liver cirrhosis mortality in 187 countries between 1980 and 2010: A systematic analysis. BMC Medicine. 2014;**12**:145. DOI: 10.1186/s12916-014-0145-y

[27] Brown GT, Kleiner DE. Histopathology of nonalcoholic fatty liver disease and nonalcoholic steatohepatitis. Metabolism. 2016;**65**(8): 1080-1086. DOI: 10.1016/j.metabol.2015.11.008

[28] Portmann BC, Roberts EA. Developmental abnormalities and liver disease in childhood. MacSween's Pathology of the Liver. 2012:101-156. DOI: 10.1016/B978-0-7020-3398-8.00003-9

[29] Toshikuni N, Tsutsumi M, Arisawa T. Clinical differences between alcoholic liver disease and nonalcoholic fatty liver disease. World Journal of Gastroenterology. 2014;**20**(26): 8393-8406. DOI: 10.3748/wjg.v20.i26.8393

[30] Aslam A, Kwo PY. Epidemiology and disease burden of alcohol associated liver disease. Journal of Clinical and Experimental Hepatology. 2023;**13**: 88-102

[31] Carr RM, Oranu A, Khungar V. Nonalcoholic fatty liver disease: Pathophysiology and management. Gastroenterology Clinics of North America. 2016;**45**(4):639-652. DOI: 10.1016/j.gtc.2016.07.003

[32] Yeh MM and Swanson PE. Hepatobiliary system. In: Gattuso P, et al. editors. Differential Diagnosis in Surgical Pathology. 2nd ed. China: Saunders Elsevier; 2012. p. 415

[33] Treseler PA, Higgins JP. Hematopoietic tumors of the liver. In: Ferrell L, Kakar S, editors. Liver Pathology. Vol. 4. New York: Demos Medical; 2011. pp. 469-491

[34] Murakami J, Shimizu Y. Hepatic manifestations in hematological disorders. International Journal of Hepatology. 2013;**2013**:484903. DOI: 10.1155/2013/484903

[35] Griscom JT, Wolf PS. Liver Metastasis. In: StatPearls [Internet]. Treasure Island (FL): StatPearls Publishing; 2023. Available from: https://www.ncbi.nlm.nih.gov/books/NBK553118 [Accessed: September 18, 2022]

[36] Asafo-Agyei KO, Samant H. Hepatocellular Carcinoma. In: StatPearls [Internet]. Treasure Island (FL): StatPearls Publishing; 2023. Available from: https://www.ncbi.nlm.nih.gov/books/NBK559177 [Accessed: February 12, 2023]

Chapter 8

Postmortem Analysis in Drowning-Related Death Determination: Application of the "Diatom Test" in the Forensic Field in Bosnia and Herzegovina

Emina Dervišević, Ermin Mašić, Muhamed Katica, Nina Čamdžić, Zurifa Ajanović, Lejla Dervišević, Muamer Dervišević, Adis Salihbegović, Suada Kuskunović-Vlahovljak and Edna Supur

Abstract

Microscopic signs are not specific only to drowning, but to any other type of suffocation, the background of which is mechanical obstruction. What about cases where there are no soft tissues when he has a skeletal body? This pilot research aims to examine for the first time the attendance of diatoms in teeth and bones, with regard to the peripheral vascularization of bones and teeth, in the Bosnia River. The thirty rats were divided into groups: Group A (n = 6; autopsy—1 hour after death; cause of death-hanging); Group B (n = 6; autopsy—72 hours after death; cause of death-hanging); Group C (n = 6; autopsy—immediately after drowning; cause of death-drowning); Group D (n = 6; autopsy—24 hours after drowning; cause of death-drowning) and Group E (n = 6; autopsy—72 hours after drowning; cause of death-drowning). In Group D and Group E, diatoms were found in one rat per group. By optimizing the "Diatom Test" in experimental settings, it could potentially become a routine method in the future. This is just the initial research that leads us toward optimizing testing and taking samples in cases of uncleared etiology, when there are no preserved soft tissue structures for autopsy.

Keywords: post-mortem, suspicious death, drowning, forensic sciences, forensic pathology

1. Introduction

The primary function of the Agency, under prescribed jurisdiction and scope, is conducted through forensic investigations and examinations in dedicated laboratories staffed with personnel trained in specialized disciplines and equipped with advanced technology, following prescribed standards for each field. According to the type of examination, the Agency has established the following laboratories:

- Laboratory for examining computer systems
- Laboratory for graphological/graphoscopic examinations
- Laboratory for examining photo and video materials
- Laboratory for examining voice and audio recordings
- Laboratory for chemical–physical examinations
- Laboratory for chemical-toxicological examinations
- Laboratory for biological examinations and DNA analysis
- Laboratory for dactyloscopy examinations

Forensic medicine in Bosnia and Herzegovina has been utilizing conventional and available laboratories for DNA and toxicological sample analysis. In the case of unexplained deaths that are sudden, abrupt, or violent, it is within the competence of the prosecutor's office to issue orders for autopsy and expert examination by an expert either singly or through designated institutes. Considering that diatom analyses are not usually used during the autopsy of drowning victims and are instead reliant on macroscopic assessments by forensic pathologists and microscopic observations, these two methods are mostly insufficient to be established as a definitive. Diatom test method, primarily, requires the development of technical and human resources and a profound knowledge of the classification of silicate algae (diatoms). Pathophysiological processes that occur during drowning have been known for a long time [1]. A fluid medium with sediment and microscopic organisms come through the initial parts of the respiratory and digestive tract and passes through the windpipe into the lungs and then through the alveoli into the circulation. The fluid with all its contents is transported to the organs by large blood flow and settles in their capillaries [2]. Diatoms as unicellular organisms remain present longer in the tissue material. Diatoms are present in freshwater habitat types. These unicellular algae can be easily isolated from organs by acid digestive extractions [3]. From then, until today, there are many conflicting opinions regarding these algae [4]. However, it is also a fact that there is no specific method for diagnosis that would help with the cause of death and the diagnosis of drowning. All types of asphyxia that arose in the background due to mechanical obstruction have nonspecific microscopic findings. Macroscopic signs of drowning on autopsy can be described as pulmonary edema and the presence of a deposit of small microscopic particles that reach the deepest parts of the respiratory system through the bronchial tree. What about situations where there are no soft tissues when he has a skeletal body?

Then, we have a bone and a tooth to identify the DNA and to determine the diatoms from them. Meanwhile, some researchers believe that the diatoms that can be found in other tissues got there from the lungs and that they could not have come through the digestive system [5]. Despite this, the diatom detection test is one of the most commonly used tests to diagnose drowning. Diatoms are a large group of algae that are present in stagnant waters as phytoplankton's. There are more than 100,000 extant species, either floating freely, plankton forms, or attached to the substrate. Diatoms are a unicellular group of organisms that are formed in almost all water bodies. They occur in the water as plankton or on the bottom where they may be attached to plants or rocks or sand particles. Diatoms are being used excessively as forensic tools for the confirmation of death due to drowning or homicide. The valve-faced diatom frustules are ornamented with pores, spines, hyline areas, and other morphological features. Diatoms are divided into two orders: (1) the central (now called the areola) which tends to appear radially symmetrical and (2) the pennales which have valve striae arranged about a line that tend to appear on both sides symetrically [6].

1.1 Forensic importance

Diatoms find varied applications in all the fields of science and technology as well as in the field of forensic science. Diatomology is the study of diatoms, and forensic diatomology is the application of diatomology in forensic science. Forensic diamotology has a crucial role in resolving unclear cases of drowning. It is crucial both to solve the source of fatal outcome and to find the place where the drowning occurred. Whether the body was brought, moved, or drowned in the same water and found. Finding diatoms in tissues can play a key role in determining drowning. The species found must correlate and match the species analyzed in the water. The diatom extraction method was improved by acid digestion of the tissue. Way back in 1949, researchers discovered the presence of diatoms in the marrow of bones. When drowning, water is inhaled, and in this way, it reaches the deeper parts of the respiratory system, leading to the expansion of the lung alveoli. These algae pass the barrier between the alveolar walls and small blood vessels and then reach the pulmonary venous blood stream. This pulmonary venous blood, full of diatoms, reaches the left atrium, and then the left heart chamber, where it spreads throughout the circulation, leading to embolization of small blood vessels in numerous organs and tissues such as bone marrow. This supports the fact that fatal drowning was a factor contributing to death and was antemortem. The main purpose of the diatom test is to differentiate death caused by drowning, from submerging an already dead body in water to conceal the actual causes of death. Diatoms are specific indicators in forensics that help medical personnel establish the actual cause of death, especially in cases where personnel are unsure of the cause of death. These algae can be found in numerous organs and tissues, such as lungs, stomach, bone marrow, and other large organs [6].

The morphological characteristics of diatoms remain well preserved even after chemical digestion, which enables forensic scientists to recognize and classify them into groups. Certain types of diatoms are a specific finding in certain types of stagnant water, which enables forensic experts to establish the place of death because suspects cannot easily hide them or remove them from the body. Although a large number of species and subspecies of diatoms are found in different aquatic diversities, this is not encountered in most cases of drowning. Given the high sensitivity to changes in the environment and living conditions, the number of diatoms can vary between different types of water media [7]. If, due to mosquito bites, diatom species from tissue and water match, this will be strong evidence and indicator that the person drowned in that particular place. Limiting factors should be taken into account when analyzing the results of diatom tests, and these test results should be analyzed together with other evidence and indicators in order to determine the cause of death as accurately as possible [8].

1.2 Diatom test

Test with the use of diatoms is a forensic technique used to determine whether a person has died by drowning [9]. In the diatom test, samples of water and tissue from the lungs and other organs of the deceased are collected and examined under a microscope to determine if diatoms are present.

However, it is important to keep in mind that the lack of diatoms in the tissue samples does not necessarily rule out drowning [9, 10]. Overall, the diatom test is just one tool in a forensic investigation and must be used in combination with other findings and data to make a conclusive resolution of the cause of death.

One of the special significances of the diatom test is its possibility to provide strong evidence of drowning when diatoms are found in the lungs but not in the surrounding water.

Despite its usefulness, the diatom test has been criticized for its limitations. For example, the test requires the collection of tissue samples, which may be difficult or impossible in certain circumstances, such as when the body has been severely decomposed or lost at sea. Additionally, diatoms can be present in water sources that are not related to drowning, leading to potential false positives [11].

In conclusion, the diatom test is a valuable forensic tool in deciding about the cause of fatal outcomes in cases of drowning, but it should be used in combination with other data and findings to make a definitive determination about the cause of fatal outcomes.

1.2.1 The positive side of the diatom test

An advantage of the test with diatoms is that it can provide strong evidence that a person has drowned by identifying the presence of diatoms in the lung tissue of the deceased. Diatoms are specific to water and have unique shapes and sizes, which means that they can be used to identify the source of water in which a person may have drowned [12].

In cases where diatoms are found in the lung tissue but not in the sample of the water medium where the body was found, there is strong evidence that the person was alive at the time of submersion and inhaled water into their lungs. This can help forensic investigators to determine the cause of death and provide important evidence for legal proceedings.

The diatom test has also been used successfully in cases where other evidence is lacking, such as when a body has been in water for an extended period or when there are no witnesses to drowning [12].

Overall, the positive side of the diatom test is that it provides a useful and scientifically valid method for determining if a person has drowned and can provide important evidence in forensic investigations.

1.2.2 The negative side of the diatom test

The negative side of the diatom test is that there are certain limitations and the possibility of error that may affect the accuracy of the results of this test.

One of the main limitations of the diatom test is that it can only provide evidence of drowning if diatoms are present in the lung tissue. If the victim does not inhale water into their lungs, the test will not provide any evidence of drowning. Additionally, the absence of diatoms in the tissue does not necessarily rule out drowning, as diatoms may not always be present or may not be preserved in the tissue due to various factors such as the length of time the body was submerged or the temperature of the water [13].

Another limitation of the diatom test is that it relies on the collection of tissue samples from the body of the deceased, which may not always be possible due to various factors such as the condition of the body or the location where it was found.

The diatom test can also be affected by potential sources of error, such as contamination of the tissue samples or the water samples used for comparison. Diatoms may also be present in bodies of water that are not related to drowning, leading to potential false positives [14, 15].

2. Methods

An experimental randomized study was conducted using the Principles for Care of Experimental Animals at the Faculty of Medicine, Veterinary Medicine and Natural Sciences of the University of Sarajevo. After the approval of the Ethics Committee of the Faculty of Medicine of the University of Sarajevo, Bosnia and Herzegovina (number: 02–3-4-AK-6589/23), a total number of 30 adult Albino rats were included in the study (body weight: 250–300 g). The drowning model developed according to knowledge and practice was used. All conditions for the care and feeding of animals ad libitum were met.

Using an experimental model of drowning, we tried for the first time in our country to investigate the presence of diatoms in teeth and bones, immediately after drowning and after 24 and 72 hours.

2.1 Experimental design

Thirty rats were divided into groups: Group A (n = 6; autopsy: 1 hour after death; cause of death: hanging); Group B (n = 6; autopsy: 72 hours after death; cause of death: hanging); Group C (n = 6; autopsy: immediately after drowning; cause of death: drowning); Group D (n = 6; autopsy: 24 hours after drowning; cause of death: drowning), and Group E (n = 6; autopsy: 72 hours after drowning; cause of death: drowning) (**Figure 1**).

In groups A and B, the cause of death was hanging; then, they were drowned in a container containing river water and taken out 1 h and 72 h after immersion. A complete examination (macroscopic, microscopic, and diatom test) was performed

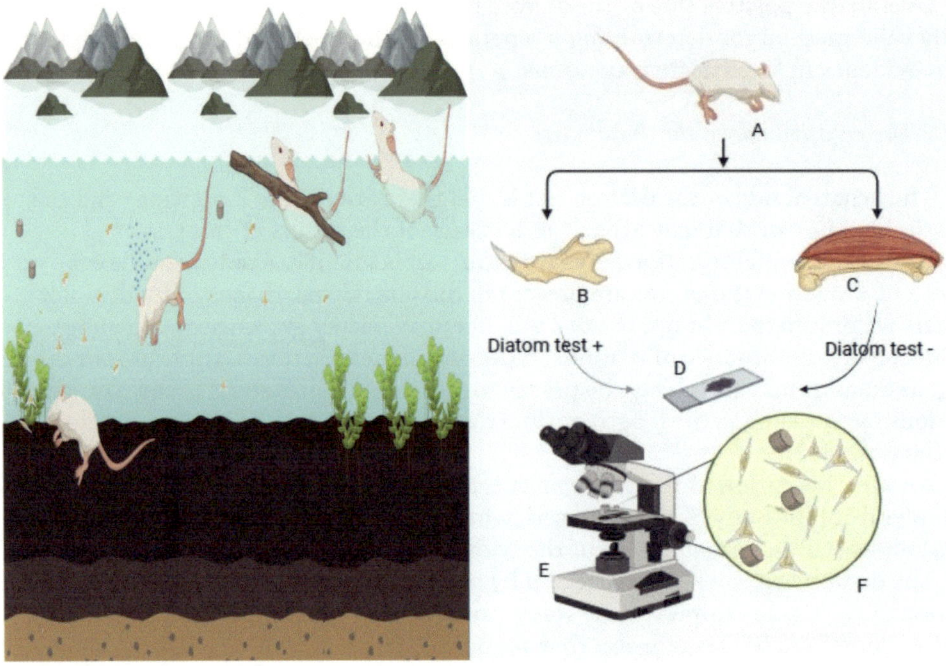

Figure 1.
Postmortem procedure for diatom isolation from tooth and bone samples (a: Rat after drowning; B: Tooth sample; C: Lat. os femur (bone); D: Suspension diatoms; E: Microscopy of diatom suspension; F: Determination of diatoms).

on each animal. Guidelines for diatom analysis were used throughout all phases of the protocol, and they have been tested from the Bosna river. Teeth and bone femur were examined samples.

2.2 Collection of phytobenthos: Study site

The "experimental crime scene" took place at the confluence of the Željeznica river with the Bosna river from the coastal part (coordinates: 43°50′28"N and 18°17′10″E at an altitude of 490 meters). During water sampling for physicochemical analysis and benthic algae, it was observed that the sky was completely cloudy and there was a light breeze. No precipitation was recorded. The water color at the time of sampling was green. Basic physicochemical parameters of the water were measured using a portable multimeter. The conductivity was 337.8 μS/cm, and water turbidity was 2.42 NTU. The pH was 7.35.

In the coastal area where the sampling was conducted, the dominant vegetation consisted of floodplain forests of the Alnetea glutinosae class, where alder (*Alnus glutinosa*) and willow (*Salix alba*) were dominant species (**Figure 2**).

After collection, the living algal material was transported to the Laboratory of the Biology Department of the University of Sarajevo. Phytobenthos samples were fixed with 4% formalin. For the laboratory approach, the method according to Hustedt [16] was used. Potassium permanganate (KMnO4), sulfuric acid (H2SO4), and oxalic acid

DOI: http://dx.doi.org/10.5772/intechopen.1004155

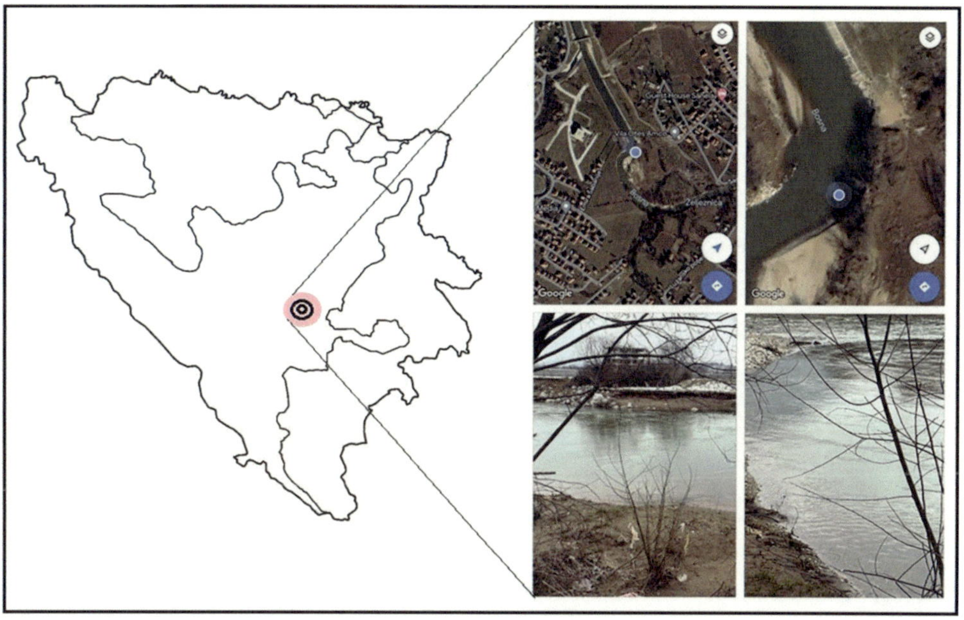

Figure 2.
Location of water and algae phytobenthos sampling.

(C2H2O4) were used for digestion. After the procedure, the cleaned diatom valves were embedded in Canadian balsam. Microscopy was performed under a magnification of 1000x (Best Scope 2020). The identification of diatoms is supported by the following references (17, 18). The methodology of the study was focused on the sampling and determination of benthic algae and monitoring the physicochemical factors of the water. Light microscope observation was conducted using the Best Scope 2020 microscope.

2.2.1 Determination of physicochemical water factors

Physicochemical factors of the water were measured immediately before the collection of benthic algae samples. Using a portable Orion Star A329 multimeter, the electrical conductivity and pH value were measured, while water turbidity was measured using a portable turbidimeter AQ3010.

3. Results

A total of 12 taxa were identified. Algae from the phyla Chlorophyta [2] and Heterokontophyta (10 taxa) dominated. The species diversity was composed of the following taxa: Nitzschia recta, *Mougeotia sp.*, Meridion circulare, *Pediastrum sp.*, *Cymbella sp.*, *Encyonema sp.*, Fragilaria vaucheriae, *Synedra ul.*, *Navicula sp.*, *Surirella sp.*, Achnanthidium minutissimum, and *Gomphonema minutum.*

Representatives of the zoobenthos were also observed in the sample: *Gammarus cf. bosniacus* and larvae of aquatic insects (genus *Baetis*) (**Figures 3–6**).

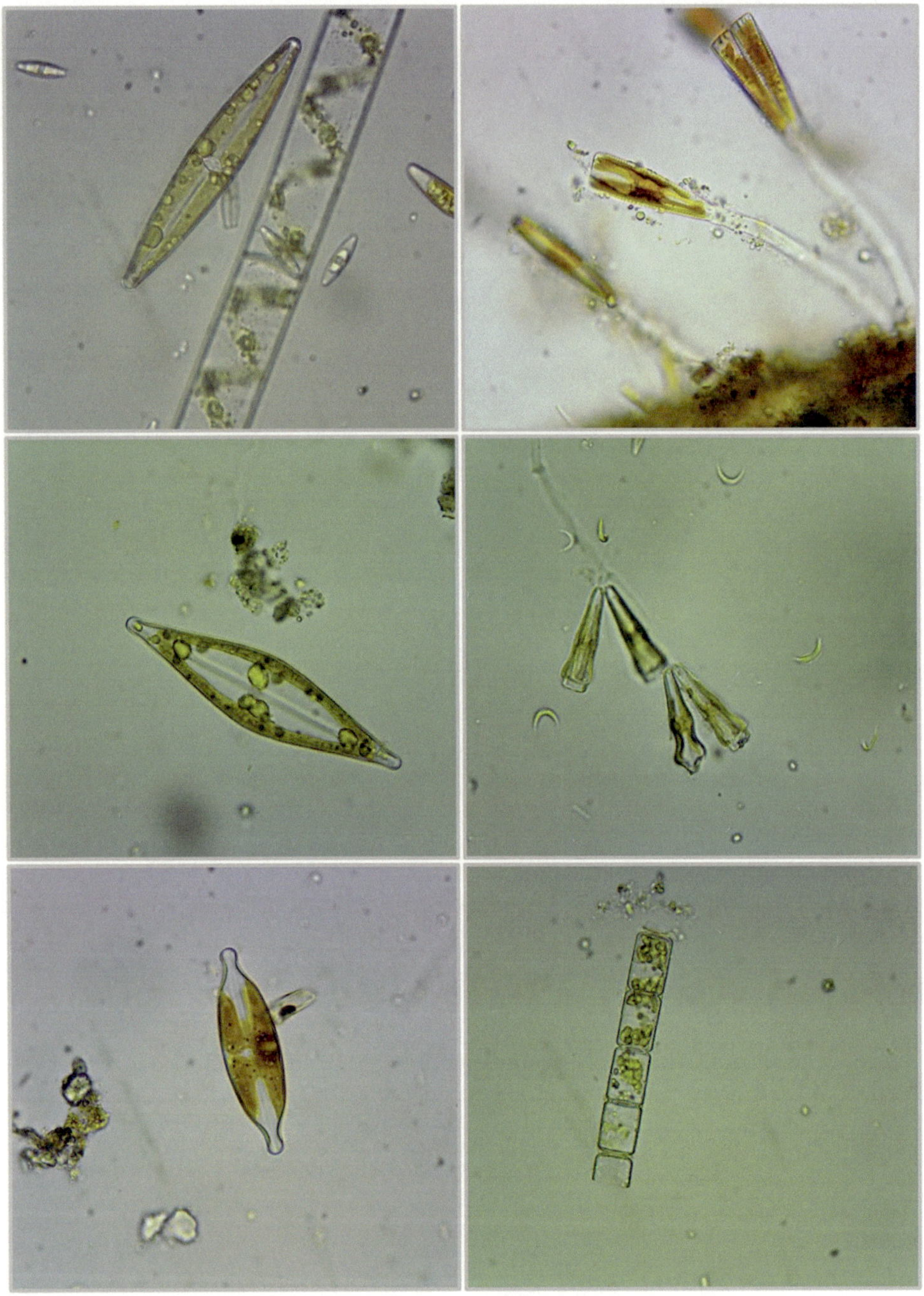

Figure 3.
Species diversity.

In Group D and Group E, diatoms were found in one rat per group, but in groups A, B, and C, no diatoms were found. The diatom test is positive when considering the tooth analysis (**Figures 7–9**).

Within all investigated groups, no diatoms were found. The diatom test is negative when considering the bone analysis.

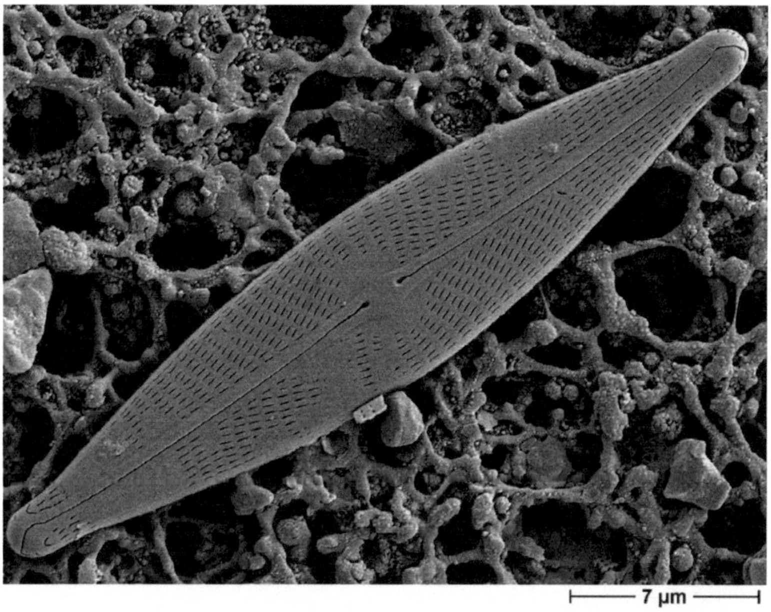

Figure 4.
Valve view of Navicula cryptocephala (SEM microphotographs).

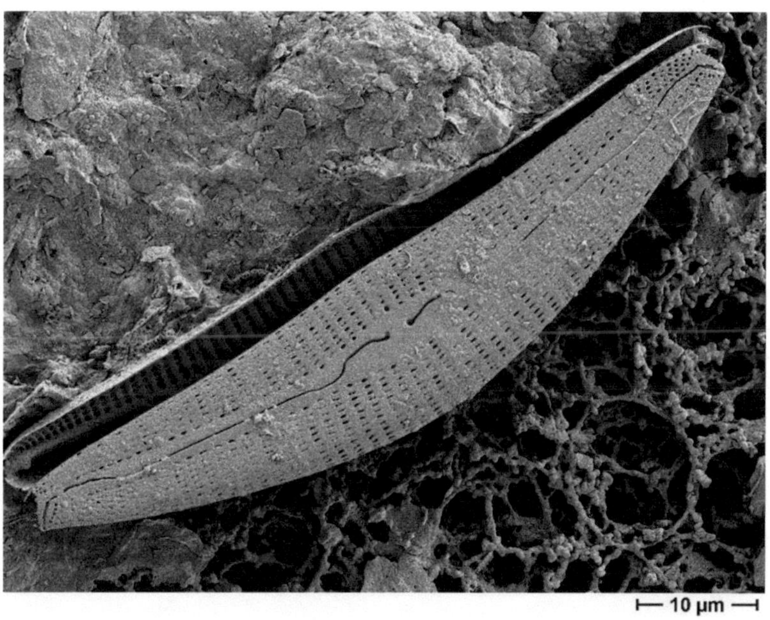

Figure 5.
Valve view of Cymbella cymbiformis (SEM microphotographs).

3.1 Comparative analysis of benthic algae in the sample and isolated parts of rats (teeth and bones)

The water sample used for experimental purposes (rat drowning in laboratory conditions) was analyzed under a light microscope (temporary and permanent

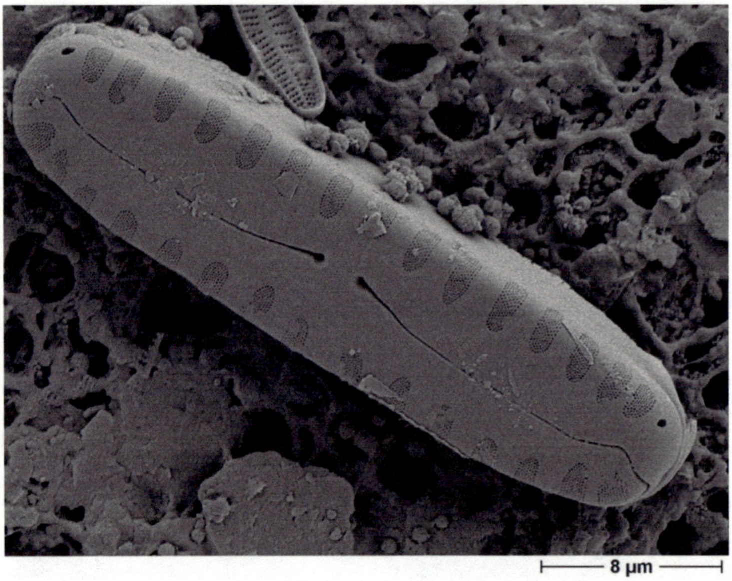

Figure 6.
Valve view of Pinnularia borealis (SEM microphotograph).

Group (Teeth)	1 RAT	2 RAT	3 RAT	4 RAT	5 RAT	6 RAT	TOTAL
A	NA	NA	NA	NA	NA	NA	NA
B	NA	NA	NA	NA	NA	NA	NA
C	-	-	-	-	-	-	-
D	-	-	-	+	-	-	+
E	-	-	-	-	-	+	+

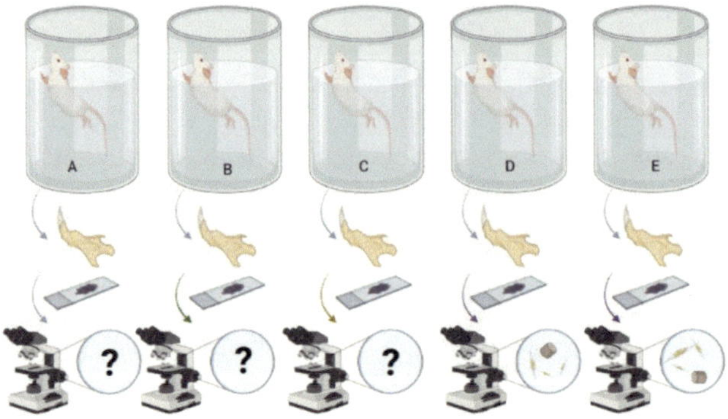

Figure 7.
Results of the diatom analysis from the tooth (positive diatom test for groups D and E). NA: Diatoms are not analyzed. -: Diatoms are not found in samples; +: Diatoms are found in samples.

slides), and the presence of several algal species was confirmed, with diatoms being among the most dominant. Within the experimental group of rats in the tooth (groups D and E), diatoms were confirmed, including *Denticula kützingii*, *Cocconeis placentula*, and *Gomphonema minutum*.

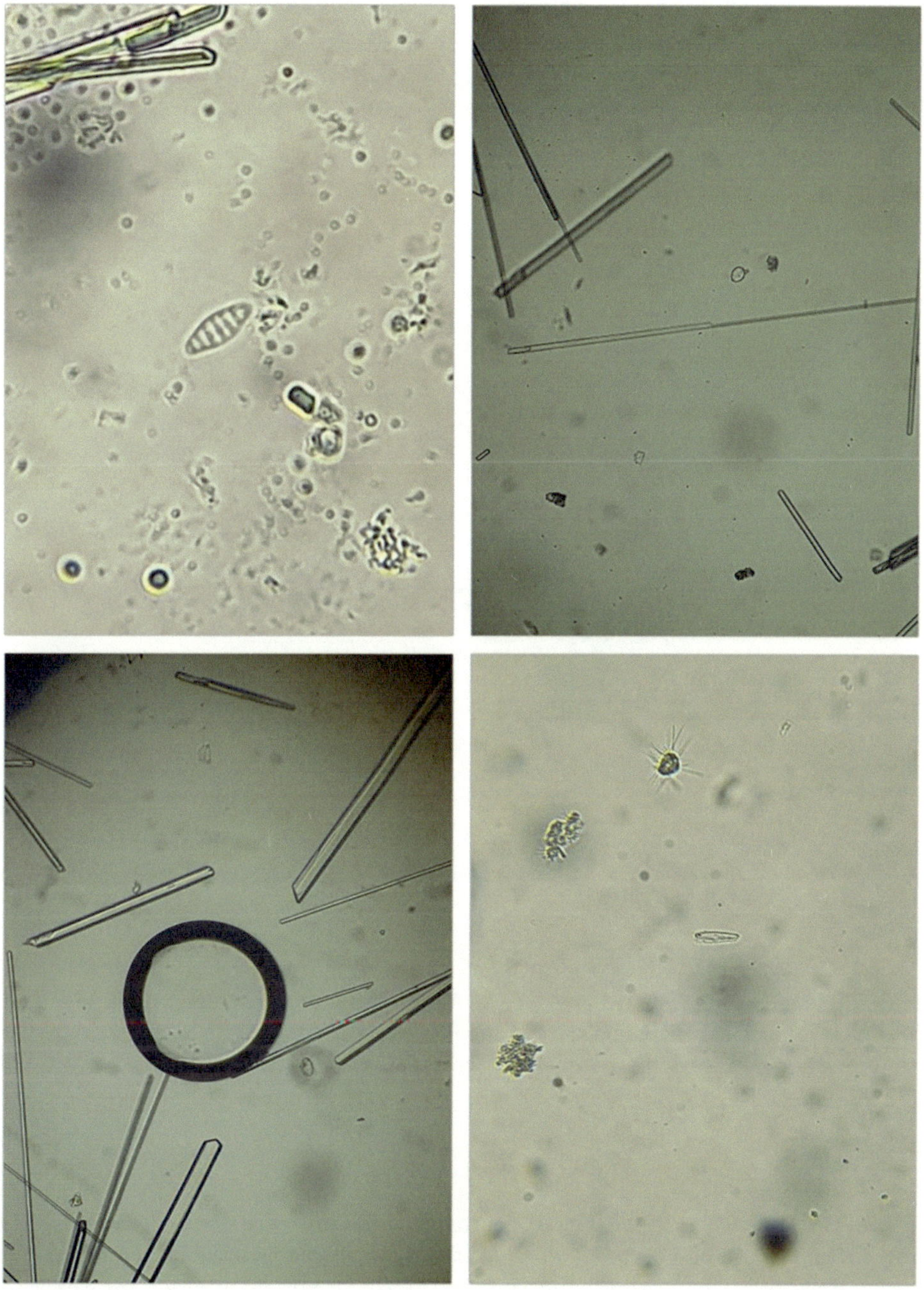

Figure 8.
Diatoms detected in the tooth (positive diatom test for groups D and E) (species detected: Denticula kützingii, Cocconeis placentula, and Gomphonema minutum).

A negative diatom test was observed within the experimental group in the bone. Diatoms were not found in any of the rats. It is important to note that the number of diatoms found in the teeth within the experimental groups D and E was extremely scarce, and the reason for this should be attributed to the quality and type of the

Group (Bone)	1 RAT	2 RAT	3 RAT	4 RAT	5 RAT	6 RAT	TOTAL
A	NA	NA	NA	NA	NA	NA	NA
B	NA	NA	NA	NA	NA	NA	NA
C	-	-	-	-	-	-	-
D	-	-	-	-	-	-	-
E	-	-	-	-	-	-	-

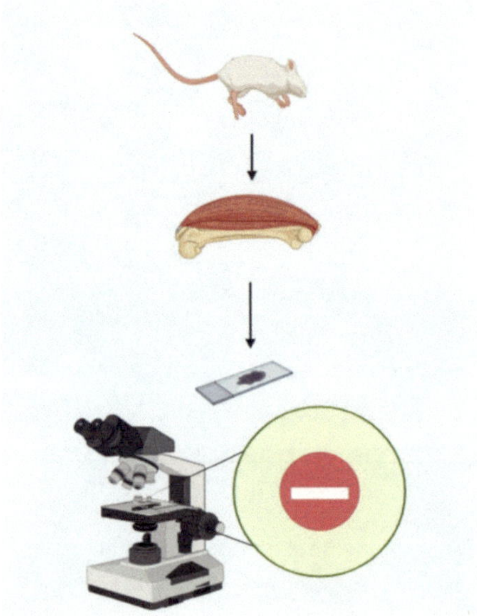

Figure 9.
Results of the diatom analysis from the bones (negative diatom test for all analyzed groups). NA: Diatoms are not analyzed. -: Diatom is not found in samples.

collected water sample. The water sample for experimental purposes was collected during the summer season and was free of mud, fine sand, detritus, and stone pebbles. Unfortunately, the quantity of algae in the phytoplankton was not significant, which is evident in the investigated samples (**Figure 10**).

4. Discussion

Whether drowning is the cause of death or the place where the body was found is just the final stage of a person's disappearance is still becoming a very interesting and completely unanswered question in forensic medicine practice. However, dead bodies in water sometimes do not have predictable marks of drowning, which makes the diagnosis of drowning tremendously controversial. Since diatoms are photoautotrophic organisms, they can enter the human body through the respiratory tract during drowning and spread through the bloodstream to all organs in the body [8–14]. Meanwhile, the presence of diatoms in the tissues can be considered a vital reaction that indirectly proves that the deceased went through the drowning process [15]. The ability of diatoms to adapt and reproduce results in large differences in the distribution of diatoms in different biodiversities. Thanks to this knowledge, the

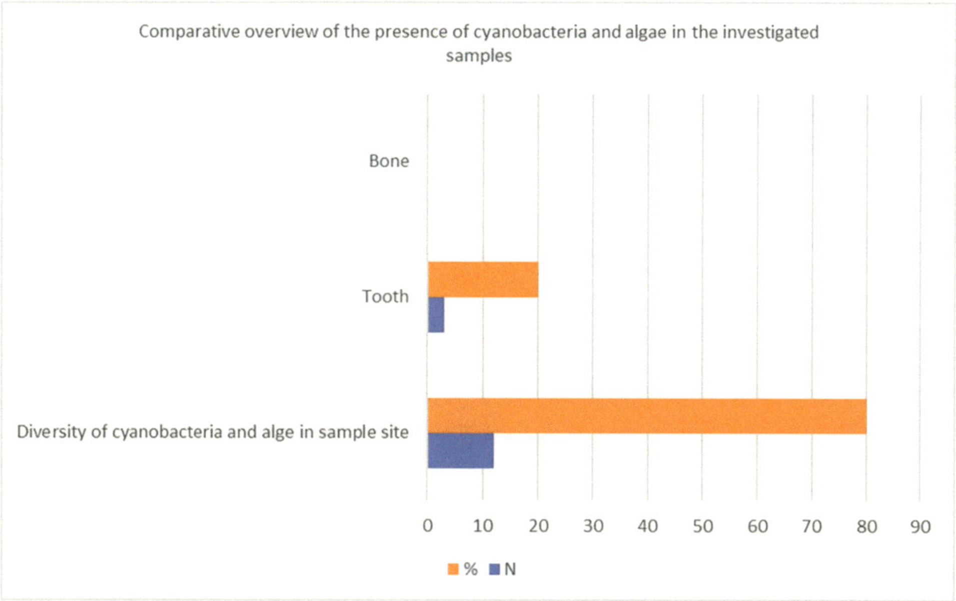

Figure 10.
Comparative representation of the presence of algae in the investigated samples.

potential determination of the place of drowning would have great forensic-medical significance. At the moment, the most common method of morphological examination is based on digestion with strong acids [16].

There are also certain limitations, which as examining a larger sample, in different parts of the year, and applying this methodology to the bodies that were pulled out of the water at the site of the investigation and examining the appearance of diatoms in the teeth. Despite all the applied methods in forensic death investigation, the use of diatoms can provide valuable support, and it is essential to consider the limitations of this method.

In river ecosystems, it is best to compare the composition of benthic algae, while in lake ecosystems, both phytoplankton and benthic algae composition can be considered.

In addition to soft tissues, for rapid screening, teeth or bones can be used. If the body has been in the water for a short time, diatoms may not reach the bones, only soft tissues and possibly teeth. Water and benthic algae sampling should follow the guidelines of the Water Framework Directive (BAS EN 15708:2011). Tissue sampling for analysis should also be optimized to minimize possible sample contamination [17–19].

Water and benthic algae, as well as phytoplankton, must be sampled by a well-trained person. The same applies to tissue sampling, preferably in laboratory conditions, using sterile equipment and adhering to safety measures for the sampler (biohazard).

5. Conclusion

The mentioned method has proven to be highly successful in assessing the location and time of drowning on a global scale, but it has not yet been widely adopted in local contexts. By optimizing the "diatom test" method in experimental settings, it could potentially become a routine method in the future. This is just the initial research that leads us toward optimizing tests in cases of unresolved etiology, when there are no preserved soft tissue structures for autopsy, and teeth and bones become available materials for diagnosing the cause of death with standardized nonspecific findings when there are no organs for micro- and macroanalysis.

Author details

Emina Dervišević[1]*, Ermin Mašić[2], Muhamed Katica[3], Nina Čamdžić[4], Zurifa Ajanović[5], Lejla Dervišević[5], Muamer Dervišević[6], Adis Salihbegović[1], Suada Kuskunović-Vlahovljak[4] and Edna Supur[7]

1 Faculty of Medicine, Department of Forensic Medicine, University of Sarajevo, Sarajevo, Bosnia and Herzegovina

2 Faculty of Science, Department of Biology, University of Sarajevo, Sarajevo, Bosnia and Herzegovina

3 Veterinary Clinical Pathology, Veterinary Faculty University of Sarajevo, Sarajevo, Bosnia and Herzegovina

4 Faculty of Medicine, Department of Pathology, University of Sarajevo, Sarajevo, Bosnia and Herzegovina

5 Faculty of Medicine, Department of Human Anatomy, University of Sarajevo, Sarajevo, Bosnia and Herzegovina

6 Clinic for Pulmonary Diseases and Tuberculosis "Podhrastovi", University of Sarajevo Clinical Centre, Sarajevo, Bosnia and Herzegovina

7 Faculty of Medicine, Department of Public Health, University of Sarajevo, Sarajevo, Bosnia and Herzegovina

*Address all correspondence to: emina.dervisevic@mf.unsa.ba

References

[1] Jian J, Wan L, Shao Y, et al. Postmortem chest computed tomography for the diagnosis of drowning: A feasibility study. Forensic Sciences Research. 2021;**6**(2):152-158

[2] Lunetta P, Penttilä A, Hällfors G. Scanning and transmission electron microscopical evidence of the capacity of diatoms to penetrate the alveolo-capillary barrier in drowning. International Journal of Legal Medicine. 1998;**111**:229-237 [PubMed] [Google Scholar]

[3] Lunetta P, Modell JH. Macroscopical, Microscopical, and Laboratory Findings in Drowning Victims. Vol. 3. New York (NY): Humana Press; 2005. pp. 3-77 [Google Scholar]

[4] Pollanen MS. Forensic Diatomology and Drowning. Amsterdam (The Netherlands): Elsevier; 1998 [Google Scholar]

[5] Saukko P, Knight B. Knight's Forensic Pathology. 4th ed. Boca Raton (FL): CRC Press; 2015 [Google Scholar]

[6] Saini P. Diatoms Can Speak. LAP LAMBERT Academic Publishing; 2019. pp. 1-69. ISBN: 978-620-0-29773-0

[7] Vanelslander B, Créach V, Vanormelingen P, et al. Ecological cological differentiation between sympatric pseudocryptic species in the esturine benthic diatom navicula phyllepta (bacillariophyceae)(1). Journal of Phycology. 2009;**45**:1278-1289 [PubMed] [Google Scholar]

[8] Lindeque PK, Bornman MS. Diatoms as a forensic tool: A review of literature and case work. Forensic Science International. 2016;**266**:251-257. DOI: 10.1016/j.forsciint.2016.06.008

[9] DePaolo JS, Gauthier JL, Thompson JP. The diatom test: A review and reappraisal. Journal of Forensic Sciences. 2005;**50**(6):1304-1311

[10] Brand U, McGeehin J, McKenzie JA. Diatom test for drowning: A necessary forensic tool? Forensic Science, Medicine, and Pathology. 2005;**1**(4):251-256

[11] Bourgault AM, Gagné P. Diatom test for drowning: A literature review. Journal of Forensic Sciences. 2014;**59**(6):1466-1471

[12] Boyer RS, Carson D. The diatom test for drowning: A reevaluation. Journal of Forensic Sciences. 2002;**47**(3):675-680

[13] Catts SV, Alvarado AM. The diagnosis of drowning: A meta-analysis of diagnostic accuracy. The American Journal of Forensic Medicine and Pathology. 2005;**26**(3):236-245

[14] Gantner NA, Lounsbury KM, Miller KW. The diatom test: A review of the literature and implications for forensic science. Journal of Forensic and Legal Medicine. 2017;**52**:77-82

[15] Padosch SA, Rothschild MA. The diatom test: A valuable tool for the forensic pathologist. American Journal of Forensic Medicine and Pathology. 2003;**24**(1):77-81

[16] Hustedt F. Bacillariophyta (Diatomae). In: Die Üsserwasser-flora Mitteleuropas. Jena: Heft 10; 1930. pp. 1-466

[17] Cantonati M, Kelly GM, Lange-Bertalot H. Freshwater benthic diatoms of Central Europe: Over 800 common species used in ecological assesment. In: English Edition with Updated Taxonomy and Added

Species. Koeltz Botanical. ISBN: 978-3-946583-06-6

[18] Guiry MD, Guiry GM. AlgaeBase. World-wide electronic publication, National University of Ireland, Galway. 2020. Availabel from: http:// www.algaebase.org; searched on 24 February 2023

[19] Dervišević E, Katica M, Mašić E, et al. Bone and tooth: Substrates for determining drowning: A new diagnostic procedure in forensic medicine practice? Legal Medicine. 2024;**66**:102366

Chapter 9

Determination of Injuries on the Bone: A Nigerian Study

Lilian Ebele Chris-Ozoko and Efe Jennifer Jaiyeoba-Ojigho

Abstract

Background: Determining injuries in relation to death have been highly imperative to forensic anthropologist since they provide clues on the norms, cultures and pattern of death of an individual. *Aim*: The study aimed at determining injuries among skeletal elements in the Anatomy Musuem of Delta State University, Abraka, Nigeria. *Methodology*: The study was crosssectional and a total of 150 bones which included the skulls, calvarium and pelvis were examined for the presence of ante, peri and postmortem injuries. Other injuries such as blunt force, sharp force and ballistic injuries were also studied. Chisquare test was used to evaluate an association between the bones and the time of injuries. Statistical assessment was done using SPSS 21 Software Version. Significance was accepted at $p < 0.05$. *Result*: The study showed that postmortem injuries was the most predominant (98%) among the bones. This was followed by perimortem and antemortem injuries (11.3, 10%). The percentages of blunt force, ballistic and sharp force were 98, 1.3 and 0.7% respectively. Further findings showed that there was no association between the bones and the nature of injuries that were observed ($p = 0.837$; 0.713). *Conclusion*: The study had shown that there are so many hidden facts from skeletal remains which can be of vital importance to forensic science.

Keywords: antermortem, perimortem, postmortem, injuries, Delta State, Nigeria

1. Introduction

Investigating bones for injuries have become a vital tool in forensic studies [1]. They can establish an individual's identity when compared with past medical records or ascertain the circumstances of death [1]. These injuries can be classified into ante-, peri- and postmortem depending on the time of occurrence [2–4]. Injuries are termed antemortem when they occur before death and are evidenced with partial or complete healing, visible at the fracture edges of bones as compared to peri-mortem injuries that show no signs of healing [1, 3, 5, 6]. Peri-mortem injuries occur at the time of death and they are distinguished in bones by the presence of fractures that interpret the cause death [1]. According to Elena [1], they are expressed by plastic deformation seen at the site of injury. Peri-mortem injuries also present a soft preponderant texture and regular outline as compared to postmortem injuries that are characterized with a rough preponderant texture and outline [1, 7–9]. It has been documented that postmortem bones have fracture patterns that are squared with sharp edges that are likely to cause enormous disintegration on dry bones [1, 7–9]. Post damages on bones classically reveal right-angled fractured margins, while those of peri-damages show obtuse or acute fracture angles [1, 7–9]. This have also been confirmed from computed tomographic scans [10]. It has also been acknowledged that injuries can also be blunt force, sharp force, ballistic and thermal [4]. This depends on the instruments that cause death at different time frame [1]. The blunt force injuries have been described as the most frequent type of injuries and they are associated with blunt objects or surfaces [1]. It must be frazzled that forensic assessment of dead bodies for injuries have now become a regular task for forensic pathologists, medical examiners and forensic anthropologists in various countries. Currently, examination of injuries includes the evaluation of ante-, peri-, or postmortem injuries, identification of injury patterns as well as possible association with certain objects. They have been limiting information on assessing injuries from remains of corpses in Nigeria, hence this study investigated them on dry bones in the Anatomy Museum of Delta State University, Abraka, Delta State Nigeria.

2. Materials and methods

The study was crosssectional and a total of 150 bones which included the skulls, calvarium and pelvis were investigated for the presence of ante-, peri- and postmortem injuries. They were also examined for other injuries such as the blunt force, sharp force and ballistic injuries. Data were represented in frequencies and percentages while a Chisquare test showed an association between bones and the time of injuries. Ethical approval for this work was obtained from the Department of Human Anatomy, Faculty of Basic Medical Sciences, Delta State University, Abraka, Delta State.

3. Results and discussions

Table 1 showed that 78.7, 11 and 10% of the bones had post-, peri- and antemortem injuries. Findings also showed that blunt force (98%), ballistic injuries (13%) and sharp force damages were observed among the investigated bones (**Table 2**). **Table 3** presented 45.3% calvariums, 10% pelvis, 44.7% skulls while **Table 4** illustrated the injuries that were present among these bones. It can be depicted from **Table 4** that 8.8, 20, 9%; 10.3, 13.3, 11.9%; 80, 66.7, 79.1% of the calvarium, pelvis and skull bones had ante-, peri- and postmortem injuries. Other injuries that were observed were blunt force, ballistic and sharp force (**Table 5**). These injuries were specific to the bones that were studied. According to **Table 5**, ballistic injuries was explicit on the skull and calvaria bones (98.5, 1.5%) while sharp force was specific to the calvarium (1.5%).

Time of injury	Frequency (%)
Antemortem	15 (10.0)
Perimortem	17 (11.3)
Postmortem	118 (78.7)
Total	150 (100.0)

Table 1.
Distribution of time of injury.

Nature of injury	Frequency (%)
Sharp force	1 (0.7)
Blunt force	147 (98.0)
Ballistic force	2 (1.3)
Total	150 (100.0)

Table 2.
Distribution of nature of injury.

Skeletal elements	Frequency (%)
Calvarium	68 (45.3)
Pelvis	15 (10.0)
Skull	67 (44.7)
Total	150 (100.0)

Table 3.
Distribution of examined skeletal elements.

Skeletal elements		Frequency	(%)
Calvarium	Antermorterm	6	8.8
	Perimorterm	7	10.3
	Postmorterm	55	80.9
	Total	68	100.0
Pelvis	Antermorterm	3	20.0
	Perimorterm	2	13.3
	Postmorterm	10	66.7
	Total	15	100.0
Skull	Antermorterm	6	9.0
	Perimorterm	8	11.9
	Postmorterm	53	79.1
	Total	67	100.0
Total		**200**	**(100.0)**

Table 4.
Distribution of examined skeletal elements based on time of injury.

Blunt force injury was noted on the calvarium (97%), pelvis and skull (100%) each respectively. Further findings showed that there was no association between injuries and the skeletal elements invested ($p = 0.837; 0.713$) (**Tables 6** and 7).

The study had shown that all bones that were studied had more postmortem damages. Features that were observed for this injury were desiccation and fragility. This could be as a result of exposure of these bones to the environment. Several authors are of the opinion that changes that occur to corpses after death are due to complex results from physicochemical and environmental processes [1, 4]. They are affected by

Skeletal elements		Frequency	(%)
Calvarium	Ballistic force	1	1.5
	Blunt force	66	97.1
	Sharp force	1	1.5
	Total	68	100.0
Pelvis	Blunt force	15	100.0
	Total	1	1.5
Skull	Ballistic force	66	98.5
	Blunt force	67	100.0
	Total	1	1.5
Total		**200**	**(100.0)**

Table 5.
Distribution of examined skeletal elements based on nature of injuries.

Skeletal elements	Nature of injury			Chi-square	Df	P-value
	Ballistic force	Blunt force	Sharp force			
Calvarium	1 (0.7)	66 (44.0)	1 (0.7)	1.442	4	0.837
Pelvis	—	15 (10.0)	—			
Skull	1 (0.7)	66 (42.0)	—			
Total	**2 (1.3)**	**147 (98.0)**	**1 (0.7)**			

Table 6.
Chi-square test of association between time of injury and nature of injury.

Skeletal elements	Time of injury			Chi-square	Df	P-value
	Antemortem	Perimortem	Postmortem			
Calvarium	6 (4.0)	7 (4.7)	55 (36.7)			
Pelvis	3 (2.0)	2 (1.3)	10 (6.7)	2.125	4	0.713
Skull	6 (4.0)	8 (5.3)	53 (35.3)			
Total	**15 (10.0)**	**17 (11.3)**	**118 (78.7)**			

Table 7.
Chi-square test of association between injury time and examined skeletal elements.

factors surrounded by the cadaver and the environment that they are kept [1, 4]. These factors influence the onset, increases the pace of post-mortem changes or impede it. The bones we observed having blunt force had an impact region, cranial and facial fractures. These evidences were highlighted by Casali *et al.* in her study on blunt force trauma carried out in Milan Italy [11]. According to these scholars, of the 307 victims studied, 40 and 30% had cranial and facial fractures [11]. Blunt force injury which was predominant from our study could be as a result of suicides, accidents, falls, described as factors associated with it [1]. This injury has been defined as one caused by a low-velocity contact resulting from a blunt surface or item [1]. According to Galloway [4], they occur as a consequence of accidents, sticks, and falls, with a diversity of broken patterns reliant on both internal and extrinsic circumstances. Features of antemortem injuries observed from this study were the presence of a poros, rounded and broken edges. This was consistent with the findings of Byers, who stated that the first signal of antemortem damage was the porosity around the fracture areas, indicative of bone activity, reabsorption, and fracture healing [12]. According to some scholars, the minor rounding or remodeling of the shattered edges, was the second trait of an antemortem harm, signifying that the damage occurred at least 7 days prior to death [2, 12–14]. Ballistic and sharp force injuries were also identified among the bones. The existence of an entry wound was seen in most of the ballistic bones from our study. This is the most prominent feature of a ballistic injury [15, 16]. The ballistic bones from this investigation also had a circumferential and radially branching fracture. A number of authors have associated ballistic injuries to the occurrence of projectiles, fractures connected with high impacts, wrecked materials found in either bone or the environment. In most instances, the presence of an entrance wound that is lesser than an exit wound also characterizes a ballistic injury [15, 16]. Sharp force injuries from our study were evidence with sharp lines around and within the bones suggestive of incised wounds. Our findings were not different from those of Thompson and Inglis who were of the opinion that this injury was marked by incisions that are gotten from tools pointed or those with marks in form of slashes [17].

4. Conclusion

It has been established that several injuries discovered on bones can be of immense value to forensic anthropologist in investigating crimes, nature of death of an individual as well as tell a people way of life because of the instruments associated with the death of an individual (**Figures 1** and **2**).

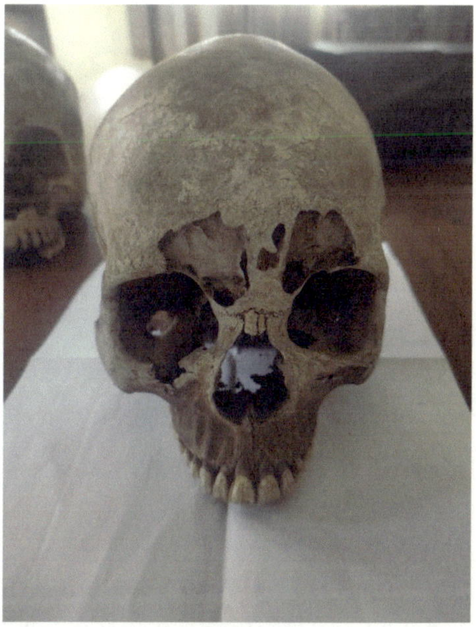

Figure 1.
A skull illustrating blunt force injury.

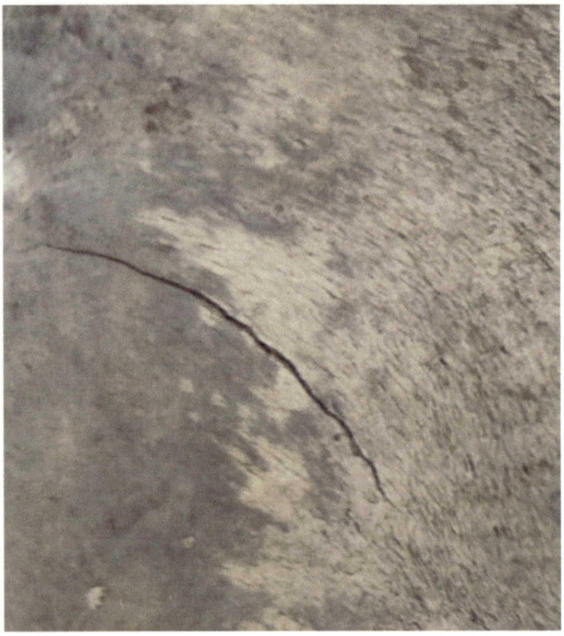

Figure 2.
A calvarium illustrating sharp force injury.

Author details

Lilian Ebele Chris-Ozoko and Efe Jennifer Jaiyeoba-Ojigho*
Faculty of Basic Medical Sciences, Department of Human Anatomy, Delta State University, Abraka, Nigeria

*Address all correspondence to: efemenadelsu@gmail.com

References

[1] Elena FK. Forensic investigation of cranial injuries due to blunt force trauma: Current best practice. Journal of Research and Reports in Forensic Medical Science. 2015;**5**:25-37

[2] Sauer N. The timing of injuries and mannerof death: Distinguishing among antemortem, perimortem, and post-mortem trauma. In: Reichs KJ, editor. Forensic Osteology: Advances in the Identification of Human Remains. 2nd ed. Springfield, IL: Charles C. Thomas; 1998. pp. 321-332

[3] Rodriguez-Martin C. Identification and differential diagnosis of traumatic lesions of the skeleton. In: Schmitt A, Cunha E, Pinheiro J, editors. Forensic Anthropology and Medicine: Complementary Sciences from Recovery to Cause of Death. New Jersey: Humana Press; 2006. pp. 197-221

[4] Galloway A. The biomechanics of fracture production. In: Galloway A, editor. Broken Bones: An Anthropological Analysis of Blunt Force Trauma. Springfield, IL: Charles C. Thomas; 1999. pp. 35-62

[5] Iscan MY, Steyn M, editors. The Human Skeleton in Forensic Medicine. 3rd ed. Springfield, IL: Charles C. Thomas; 2013

[6] Lovell NC. Trauma analysis in paleopathology. Yearbook Physical Anthropology. 1997;**40**:139-170

[7] Dirkmaat DC, Cabo LL, Ousley SD, Symes SA. New perspectives in forensic anthropology. Yearbook Physical Anthropology. 2008;**51**:33-52

[8] Morlan RE. Toward the definition of criteria for the recognition of artificial bone alterations. Quaternary Research. 1984;**22**:160-171

[9] Fleming-Farrell D, Michailidis K, Karantanas A, Roberts N, Kranioti EF. Virtual assessment of perimortem and postmortem blunt force cranial trauma. Forensic Science International. 2013;**229**(1-3):162.e1-162.e6

[10] Bonnichsen R. Pleistocene Bone Technology in the Beringian Refugium. National Museum of Man Mercury Series, Archaeological Survey of Canada Paper No 89. Ottawa, Canada; 1979

[11] Casali MB, Battistini A, Blandino A, Cattaneo C. The injury pattern in fatal suicidal falls from a height: An examination of 307 cases. Forensic Science International. 2014;**244**:57

[12] Byers SN. Introduction to Forensic Anthropology: A Textbook. 2nd ed. Pearson Education: Boston, MA; 2005

[13] Aufderheide AC, Rodriguez-Martin C. The Cambridge Encyclopedia of Human Paleopathology. Cambridge: Cambridge University Press; 1998

[14] Konstantinos M, Chara S. Identification and differentiation diagnosis of perimortem blunt force trauma in tubular long bones. Forensic Science Medical Pathology. 2006;**2**(4):221-230

[15] Smith OC, Pope EJ, Symes SA. Look until you see: Identification of trauma in skeletal material. In: Steadman DW, editor. Hard Evidence: Case Studies in Forensic Anthropology. Upper Saddle River, NJ: Prentice Hall; 2003. pp. 138-154

[16] Berryman HE, Symes SA. Recognizing gunshot and blunt cranial

trauma through fracture interpretation. In: Reichs KJ, editor. Forensic Osteology: Advances in the Identification of Human Remains. Springfield, IL: Charles C. Thomas; 1998. pp. 333-352

[17] Thompson TJU, Inglis J. Differentiation of serrated and non-serrated blades from stab marks in bone. International Journal of Legal Medicine. 2009;**123**(2):129-135

Chapter 10

Coronary Atherosclerosis: A Neglected Cause of Sudden Cardiac Death in the Young

Gaetano Thiene, Stefania Rizzo and Cristina Basso

Abstract

Sudden cardiac death (SCD) in the adult-elderly population is mostly arrhythmic due to acute thrombotic coronary artery occlusion or chronic ischemic heart disease. In the young atherosclerotic coronary artery disease (CAD) is thought to play a negligible role. We reviewed our pathology experience (1980–2016) in 690 consecutive SCDs in the young (≤40 years old, sudden infant death excluded). We found that CAD was the major cause of SCD (18%). It was observed in 125 subjects (mean age 32.3 ± 5.3 years, female 14), with a peak in 31–40 years old age interval. Site, extent, and histologic type of CAD were peculiar: single plaque of the proximal left anterior descending coronary artery, consisting of fibrocellular proliferation, with rare lipid core. The culprit atherosclerotic segment showed critical stenosis in 66% of cases and thrombotic occlusion in 34%, the latter as the consequence of plaque rupture in 47% and plaque erosion in 53%, which occurred even upon noncritical stenosis. An overt histologically acute myocardial infarction was never seen. When SCD took place during Holter monitory, transient myocardial ischemia was recorded, followed by ventricular fibrillation at the time of reperfusion. Atherosclerotic CAD was found to be the major cause of SCD also in the young, precipitated by acute coronary thrombosis in only a third of cases, more frequently upon endothelial erosion. Functional plaque instability with vasospasm, superimposed to a critical coronary plaque with ECG transient myocardial ischemia, was observed to precipitate SCD.

Keywords: atherosclerosis, coronary artery disease, epidemiology, prevention, sudden death in the young

1. Introduction

Sudden cardiac death (SCD) is a fatal event, also occurring in the young. It may be due to structural heart disease or may occur in normal hearts in the setting of Channelopathies ("mors sine materia") [1, 2]. While atherosclerotic coronary artery disease (CAD) is the most frequent cause of SCD in the adult-elderly [3–8], in the young it is considered a rare morbid entity, a belief that does not correspond to herein reported pathological experience.

 IntechOpen

2. Material and methods

In 1980 we implemented a prospective postmortem research project on sudden death in the young (age interval 2–40 years), studying all cases occurring in the Veneto Region, Italy. Most of the autopsies were carried out in peripheral hospitals.

Up to 2016, we studied 690 consecutive SCDs. The formalin-fixed heart specimens were forwarded to the Cardiovascular Pathology Unit of the University of Padua for examination, according to a thorough protocol [1, 9]. Molecular autopsy in apparently normal hearts was introduced in 2000 [10], and toxicology was performed when indicated [11]. After inspecting coronary ostia and excluding coronary artery anomalies, sections by the scalpel of the subepicardial coronary arteries were performed every 1–2 mm, and samples were formalin-fixed and paraffin-embedded for histology and immunohistochemistry.

3. Results

Sudden cardiac death was ascribed to atherosclerotic CAD in 125 out of 690 (18%) SCDs (mean age 32.3 ± 5.3, female 14). A single atherosclerotic plaque was found located in the proximal-middle tract of the left anterior descending coronary artery (LDA) in the great majority (95%).

Figure 1 reports the various causes of SCD. Atherosclerotic CAD ranks first (18%), followed by "normal heart" (17%), myocarditis (12%), arrhythmogenic cardiomyopathy (10%), hypertrophic cardiomyopathy (9%) and mitral valve prolapse (8%).

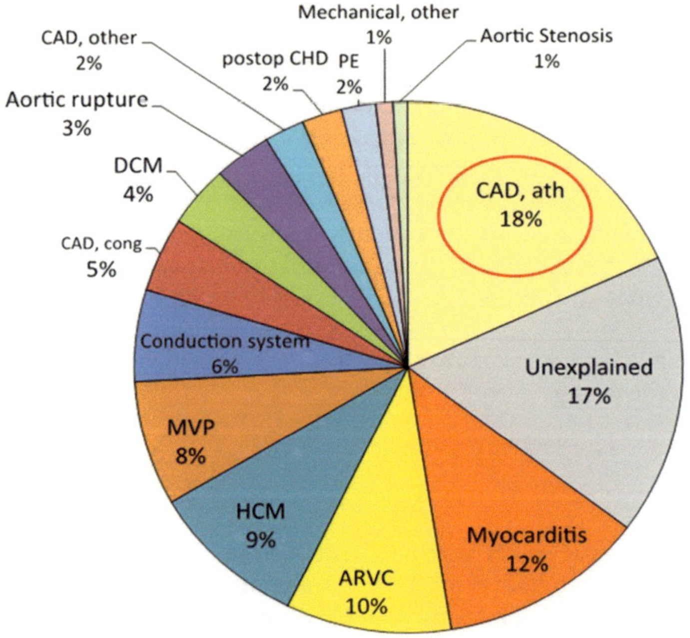

Figure 1.
Causes of sudden cardiac death in 690 young subjects, Veneto region, Italy (1980–2016). Atherosclerotic coronary artery disease (CAD) ranks first (18%). ARVC = Arrhythmogenic right ventricular cardiomyopathy; ath = atherosclerotic; CAD = coronary artery disease; cong = congenital; DCM = dilated cardiomyopathy; HCM = hypertrophic cardiomyopathy; MVP = mitral valve prolapse; postop CHD = postoperative congenital heart disease.

Figure 2 reports the various causes of SCD in 75 athletes, all male: arrhythmogenic cardiomyopathy ranks first (27%), atherosclerotic CAD second (24%), and coronary artery anomalies third (17%).

The culprit plaque in SCD by atherosclerotic CAD was either eccentric or concentric. In subjects aged less than 30 years, the plaques rarely disclosed a necrotic core ("atheroma") and were mostly fibrous, with evidence of recent intimal proliferation on the lumen side (**Figure 3**). Critical stenosis (>75%), without evidence of fresh mural or occlusive thrombosis, was observed in 76 cases (61%). In two of the latter cases, SCD occurred during Holter monitoring, with evidence of transient ST-segment elevation, turning into ventricular fibrillation during reperfusion (**Figure 3**) [12].

Thrombotic coronary artery occlusion was observed in 49 cases (39%). Plaque with fibrous cap rupture (**Figure 4**) accounted for thrombosis in 23 cases (47%, all >30 years old) and plaque erosion in 26 (53%) (**Figure 5**). The latter occurred upon noncritical plaque in 3 (**Figure 6**). Inflammatory infiltrates with endothelial disruption [13] accounted for erosion in three cases (**Figure** 7). Atherosclerotic plaques never exhibited calcification.

As far as the myocardium, histological evidence of an acute myocardial infarction was never observed, whereas fibrotic myocardial scars, in keeping with previous infarcts [1], were seen in 27% of SCD by atherosclerotic CAD.

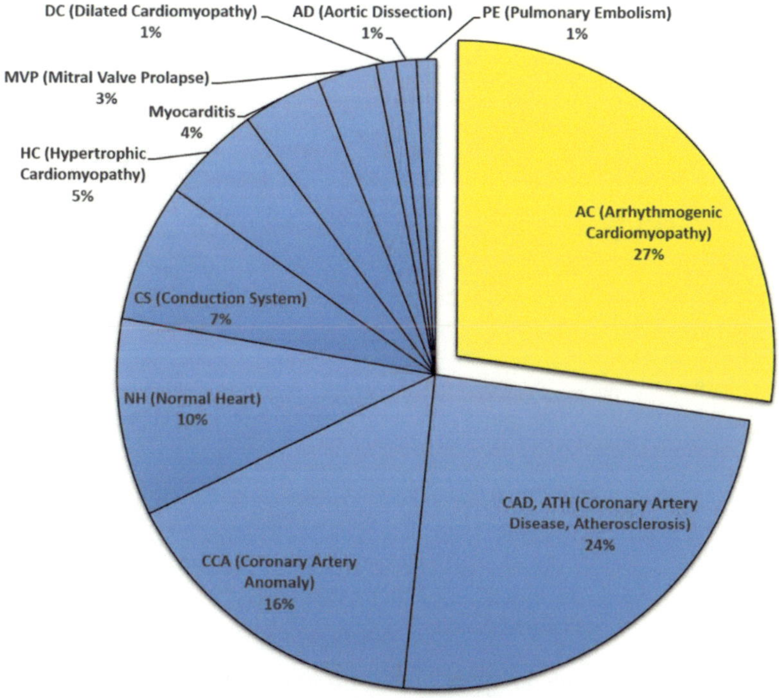

Figure 2.
Sudden cardiac death in 75 athletes. Veneto region, Italy, 1980–2016. Atherosclerotic coronary artery disease ranks second (24%). AC = Arrhythmogenic cardiomyopathy; AD = aortic dissection; CAD, ATH = coronary artery disease, atherosclerosis; CCA = coronary artery anomalies; CS = conduction system abnormalities; DC = dilated cardiomyopathy; HC = hypertrophic cardiomyopathy; MVP = mitral valve prolapse; NH = Normal heart; PE = pulmonary embolism.

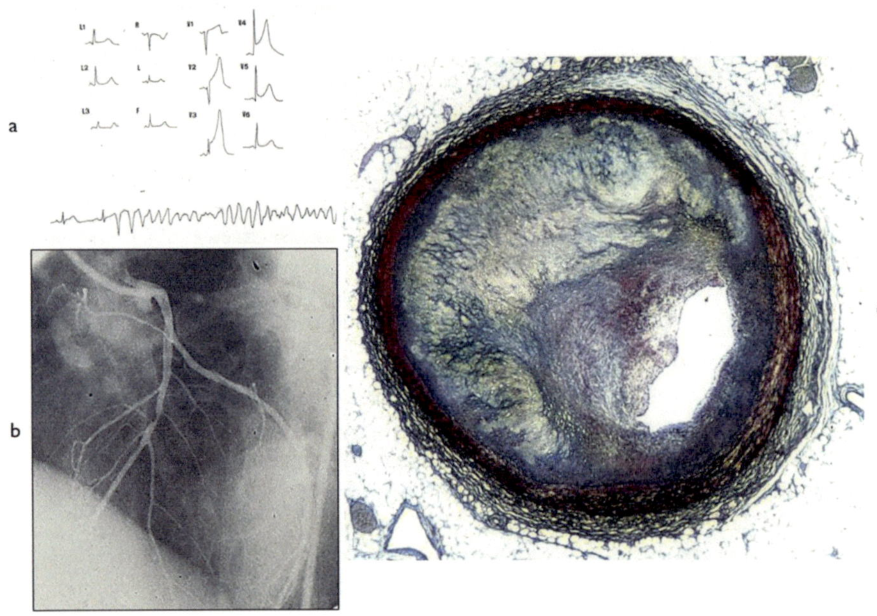

Figure 3.
Vasospasm as a cause of SCD in a young. (a) ECG with transient ischemia turning into ventricular fibrillation; (b) selective coronary artery angiography: single eccentric obstructive plaque is located in the middle tract of the anterior descending coronary artery; (c) the corresponding histology of the plaque: Fibro cellular type without atheroma, with a recent intimal proliferation (Azan Mallory stain). From [12], modified.

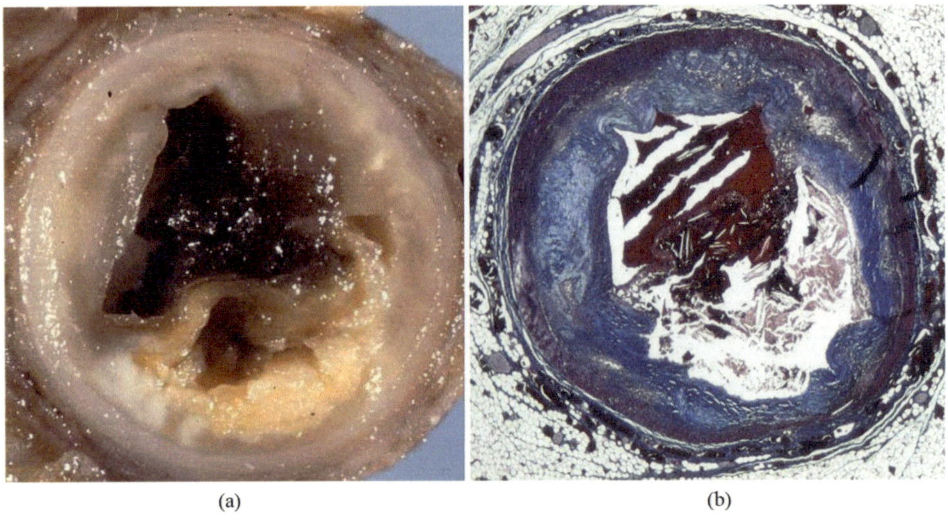

Figure 4.
Example of thrombotic occlusion by fibrous cap rupture. (a) Gross view; (b) corresponding histology. Note the disruption of the thin fibrous cap upon a large atheroma, including needles of cholesterol. Azan Mallory stain.

DOI: http://dx.doi.org/10.5772/intechopen.1002518

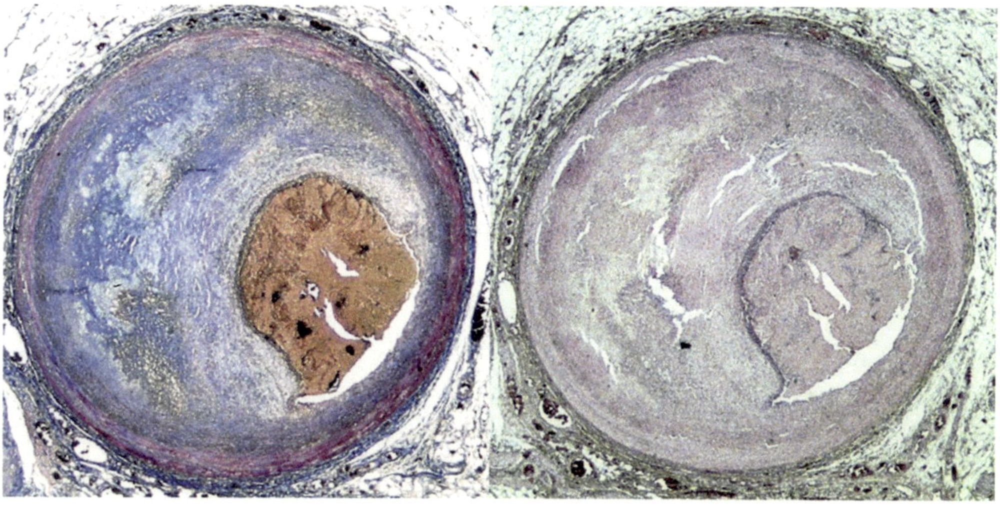

a b

Figure 5.
Endothelial erosion, complicated by thrombotic occlusion of the lumen, in an eccentric atherosclerotic plaque of the anterior descending coronary artery, with critical stenosis. (a) Azan Mallory; (b) hematoxylin–eosin. Note the subendothelial inflammatory infiltrate covering the plaque, free from atheroma.

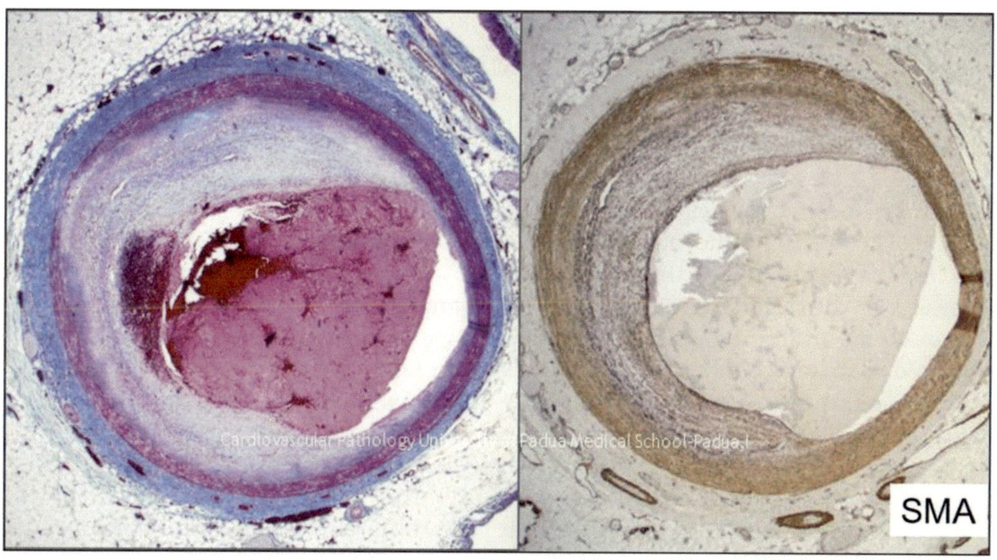

(a) (b)

Figure 6.
Erosion occlusive thrombus upon a noncritical atherosclerotic plaque, free from atheroma. (a) Hematoxylin–eosin. (b) CD 38 immunostain.

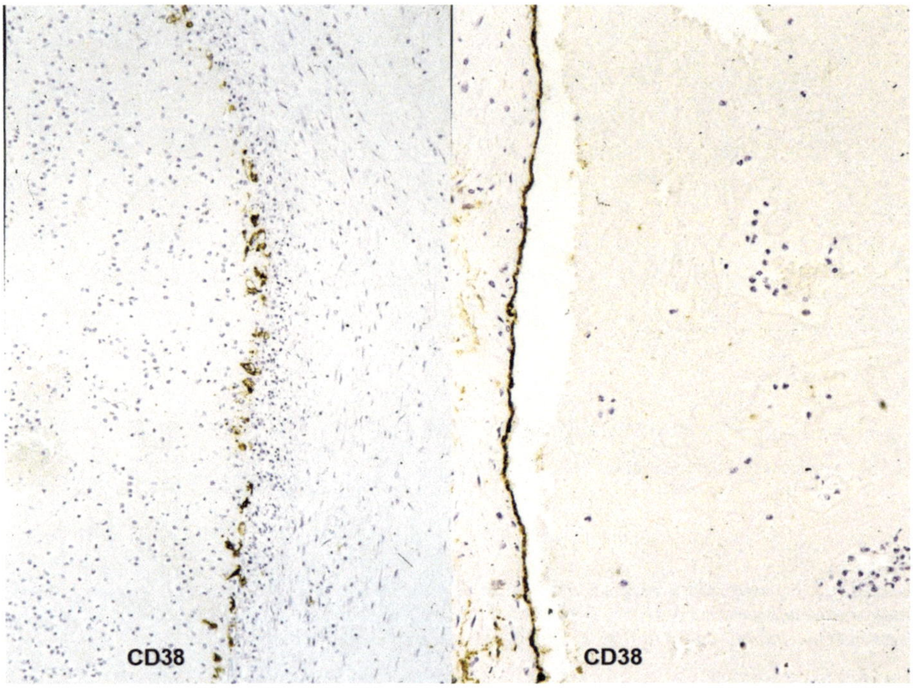

(a) (b)

Figure 7.
Occlusive coronary thrombus by erosion. (a) Inflammatory disruption of the endothelial lining at the plant base of the thrombus; (b) intact endothelial lining of the opposite side. CD 38 immunostaining.

4. Discussion

Our prospective investigation on SD in the young revealed that in the Veneto Region of Italy CAD is the major cause of SCD also in the young (2–40 years old).

CAD is a nightmare, confirming that atherosclerosis is an acquired "malignant" disease with the risk of premature SCD in the young [14]. The results of our investigation resemble an "Italian" paradox because the high rate of CAD in SCD of the young occurred in Italy, a country with a Mediterranean healthy diet.

Previous studies on the hearts of young people, who died of noncardiovascular disease, revealed that coronary atherosclerosis may appear under the age of 20 [15].

The atherosclerotic plaques of young subjects under 30 years old did not exhibit the classical characteristic of necrotic core and fibrous cap [9, 15]. They appeared fibrous, with recent intimal smooth muscle cell proliferation. Whether this is another type of arteriosclerosis or an early stage of plaque with atheroma remains elusive.

We had indeed the serendipity to study two cases who died suddenly during Holter monitoring after transient ST segment elevation [12]. A single coronary obstructive plaque was located at the proximal anterior descending coronary artery (called the coronary artery of sudden death by German pathologists). The plaque appeared either concentric or eccentric, without atheroma and fibrous cap. The ECG recorded anterior ST-segment elevation in keeping with transmural myocardial ischemia, which returned to normal in a few minutes, followed by the onset of ventricular fibrillation. Most likely, the malignant life-threatening electrical instability occurred

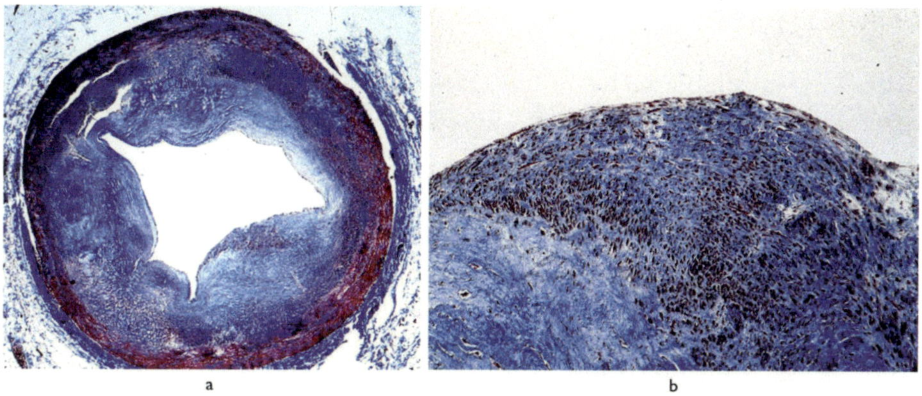

Figure 8.
A solitary plaque at the anterior descending coronary artery. (a) Panoramic view: Note the fibrocellular plaque. Azan Mallory stain; (b) close-up of the recent intimal smooth muscle cell proliferation. Hematoxylin–eosin stain.

during reperfusion at the time of spontaneous reopening of the coronary lumen. Unfortunately, the patients were alone, so resuscitation maneuvers could not be performed. At the microscope, the atherosclerotic plaques showed a recent intimal proliferation of smooth muscle cells (**Figures 3** and **8**). The tunica media appeared well preserved with normal thickness all around the coronary segment. Immunostaining demonstrated that intimal cell proliferation consisted of both synthetic and contractile smooth muscle cells, which most probably contributed to vasospasm [16]. There was no evidence of plaque rupture with platelets or fibrin adhesion. Thus cell proliferation was not consistent with plaque healing.

The origin of these subendocardial smooth muscle cells (**Figure 8**) is intriguing [17–20]. Endothelial-to-mesenchymal transition has been postulated [21].

Our findings suggest that plaque instability in the young is caused not only by plaque rupture or endothelial erosion with thrombosis but also by vasospasm of the culprit segment by intimal smooth muscle cell proliferation with contractile phenotype.

Coronary thrombosis in SCD of the young was mostly precipitated by endothelial erosion, with evidence of inflammatory disruption of the endothelium [13]. The cause of the latter is obscure. Moreover, thrombosis by erosion may occur even upon a noncritical plaque. It makes it impossible to detect by the stress test, which in Italy is mandatory for sports eligibility.

In conclusion, even in the young, atherosclerotic CAD is the main cause of SCD. Plaque instability may be either structural by thrombosis, mostly due to inflammatory erosion, or functional due to contractile intimal smooth muscle cell proliferation upon the plaque, accounting for transient coronary occlusion and acute myocardial ischemia, turning into ventricular fibrillation.

5. Limitation of the study

Data on risk factors, like smoking, cholesterol, hypertension, and familiarity, were unavailable since, in this young population, SCD occurred as a first manifestation of the disease in the absence of files from previous health visits.

Acknowledgements

This study was supported by the Registry of Cardio-Cerebro-Vascular Pathology, Veneto Region, Venice, and by ARCA Foundation, Padua, Italy.

Conflict of interest

The authors declare no conflict of interest.

Acronyms and abbreviations

CAD	coronary artery disease
ECG	electrocardiogram
LDA	left anterior descending
SCD	sudden cardiac death
SD	sudden death

Author details

Gaetano Thiene*, Stefania Rizzo and Cristina Basso
Department of Cardiac-Thoracic-Vascular Sciences and Public Health, Cardiovascular Pathology Unit, University of Padua, Padua, Italy

*Address all correspondence to: gaetano.thiene@unipd.it

References

[1] Thiene G, Corrado D, Basso C. Sudden Cardiac Death in the Young and Athletes. Text Atlas of Pathology and Clinical Correlates. Milan, Italy: Springer-Verlag; 2016. p. 190. ISBN 978-88-470-5775-3

[2] Thiene G. Sudden cardiac death and cardiovascular pathology: From anatomic theater to double helix. The American Journal of Cardiology. 2014;**114**(12):1930-1936. DOI: 10.1016/j.amjcard.2014.09.037

[3] Lovegrove T, Thompson P. The role of acute myocardial infarction in sudden cardiac death – A statistician's nightmare. American Heart Journal. 1978;**96**(6):711-713. DOI: 10.1016/0002-8703(78)90002-9

[4] Davies MJ. Stability and instability: Two faces of coronary atherosclerosis. The Paul Dudley White Lecture 1995. Circulation. 1996;**94**(8):2013-2020. DOI: 10.1161/01.cir.94.8.2013

[5] Davies MJ. Anatomic features in victims of sudden coronary death. Coronary artery pathology. Circulation. 1992;**85**(1 Suppl):I19-I24

[6] Arbustini E, Grasso M, Diegoli M, Pucci A, Bramerio M, Ardissino D, et al. Coronary atherosclerotic plaques with and without thrombus in ischemic heart syndromes: A morphologic, immunohistochemical, and biochemical study. The American Journal of Cardiology. 1991;**68**(7):36B-50B. DOI: 10.1016/0002-9149(91)90383-v

[7] Libby P. Mechanisms of acute coronary syndromes and their implications for therapy. The New England Journal of Medicine. 2013;**368**(21):2004-2013. DOI: 10.1056/NEJMra1216063

[8] Crea F, Libby P. Acute coronary syndromes: The way forward from mechanisms to precision treatment. Circulation. 2017;**136**(12):1155-1166. DOI: 10.1161/CIRCULATIONAHA.117.029870

[9] Corrado D, Basso C, Poletti A, Angelini A, Valente M, Thiene G. Sudden death in the young. Is acute coronary thrombosis the major precipitating factor? Circulation. 1994;**90**(5):2315-2323. DOI: 10.1161/01.cir.90.5.2315

[10] Basso C, Carturan E, Pilichou K, Rizzo S, Corrado D, Thiene G. Sudden cardiac death with normal heart: Molecular autopsy. Cardiovascular Pathology. 2010;**19**(6):321-325. DOI: 10.1016/j.carpath.2010.02.003

[11] Montisci M, Thiene G, Ferrara SD, Basso C. Cannabis and cocaine: A lethal cocktail triggering coronary sudden death. Cardiovascular Pathology. 2008;**17**(5):344-346. DOI: 10.1016/j.carpath.2007.05.005

[12] Corrado D, Thiene G, Buja GF, Pantaleoni A, Maiolino P. The relationship between growth of atherosclerotic plaques, variant angina and sudden death. International Journal of Cardiology. 1990;**26**(3):361-367. DOI: 10.1016/0167-5273(90)90095-m

[13] van der Wal AC, Becker AE, van der Loos CM, Das PK. Site of intimal rupture or erosion of thrombosed coronary atherosclerotic plaques is characterized by an inflammatory process irrespective of the dominant plaque morphology. Circulation. 1994;**89**(1):36-44. DOI: 10.1161/01.cir.89.1.36

[14] Thiene G. More basic research on atherosclerosis to find targeted therapy and improve prevention. Circulation.

2013;**128**:f54. DOI: 10.1161/CIR.0b013e3182a87d8aCirculation

[15] Angelini A, Thiene G, Frescura C, Baroldi G. Coronary arterial wall and atherosclerosis in youth (1-20 years): A histologic study in a northern Italian population. International Journal of Cardiology. 1990;**28**(3):361-370. DOI: 10.1016/0167-5273(90)90320-5

[16] Rizzo S, Coen M, Sakic A, De Gaspari M, Thiene G, Gabbiani G, et al. Sudden coronary death in the young: Evidence of contractile phenotype of smooth muscle cells in the culprit atherosclerotic plaque. International Journal of Cardiology. 2018;**264**:1-6. DOI: 10.1016/j.ijcard.2018.02.096

[17] Lambert J, Jørgensen HF. Vascular smooth muscle cell phenotypic switching and plaque stability: A role for CHI3L1. Cardiovascular Research. 2021;**117**(14):2691-2693. DOI: 10.1093/cvr/cvab099

[18] Miano JM, Fisher EA, Majesky MW. Fate and state of vascular smooth muscle cells in atherosclerosis. Circulation. 2021;**143**(21):2110-2116. DOI: 10.1161/CIRCULATIONAHA.120.049922

[19] Tavora F, Cresswell N, Li L, Ripple M, Fowler D, Burke A. Sudden coronary death caused by pathologic intimal thickening without atheromatous plaque formation. Cardiovascular Pathology. 2011;**20**(1):51-57. DOI: 10.1016/j.carpath.2009.08.004

[20] Horita A, Kurata A, Ohno S, Shimoyamada H, Saito I, Kamma H, et al. Immaturity of smooth muscle cells in the neointima is associated with acute coronary syndrome. Cardiovascular Pathology. 2015;**24**(1):26-32. DOI: 10.1016/j.carpath.2014.09.003

[21] Jackson AO, Zhang J, Jiang Z, Yin K. Endothelial-to-mesenchymal transition: A novel therapeutic target for cardiovascular diseases. Trends in Cardiovascular Medicine. 2017;**27**(6):383-393. DOI: 10.1016/j.tcm.2017.03.003

Chapter 11

Forensic Science: Revealing the Clues

Vaishali Abrol

Abstract

Forensic science is the discipline concerned with the systematic examination and interpretation of evidence obtained from crime scenes, employing a range of scientific methodologies. The field of forensic science comprises a range of specialised sub-disciplines within the field of criminal investigation plays a distinct role in the complex process of piecing together evidence, contributing to the creation of a cohesive narrative. In the field of forensic medicine, the significance of forensic science is further accentuated. The field of forensic science is of greatest importance in the context of postmortem examinations, as these examinations are carried out with the primary objective of determining the cause and manner of death in deceased individuals. Autopsies, which are fundamental to the field of forensic medicine, are performed in order to determine the physiological and pathological characteristics of a deceased individual. Forensic pathologists, in conjunction with forensic scientists, engage in thorough examinations utilising a variety of equipment, including microscopes, advanced imaging techniques, digital histopathological techniques, leveraging their substantial medical expertise. The collaboration between multiple disciplines ensures a holistic comprehension of the deceased individual's state, revealing key observations regarding the factors that contributed to their death. The chapter will be describing the significance of "Forensic Science" in the field of forensic medicine and its future scope.

Keywords: forensic science, forensic medicine, postmortem examination, pathology, advanced imaging technologies

1. Introduction

As a multifaceted subject that exists at the intersection of science and criminal justice, forensic science plays an important part in the process of investigating crimes and bringing victims the justice they deserve. Forensic science is the application of scientific principles and methods to the investigation of crime and the administration of justice [1]. Forensic science comprises a broad spectrum of disciplines and use scientific methodologies and procedures to analyse and interpret evidence in the context of criminal investigations and judicial proceedings. The basic objective of forensic science is to collect, examine, and evaluate tangible evidence in order to establish factual information or offer expert testimony within the context of legal processes. Forensic science encompasses a diverse array of scientific disciplines and plays a crucial role in the resolution of criminal cases, examination of evidence recovered from autopsies, the identification of potential perpetrators, and the maintenance of a fair and just legal system. The history of forensic science reflects the continuous development of techniques and methods for solving crimes, identifying victims, and ensuring justice. It has transformed from rudimentary practices into a highly specialised and multidisciplinary field that plays an indispensable role in modern criminal investigations and the legal system. During the Middle Ages in Europe, methods of trial by ordeal, such as dunking or firewalking, were used to determine guilt or innocence. The concept of "forensic medicine" began to emerge with the work of early medical practitioners, who conducted post-mortem examinations to establish causes of death [2]. The field of forensic science is of greatest importance in the context of postmortem examinations, as these examinations are carried out with the primary objective of determining the cause and manner of death in deceased individuals. Postmortem examinations, commonly referred to as autopsies, play a pivotal role in resolving inquiries pertaining to suspicious deaths, accidents, mysterious death, and various forensic investigations by providing a wide range of tools and techniques that can be used to assist forensic pathologists in their work [2]. Forensic pathologists are physicians with specialised training in the investigation of death, and they perform postmortem examinations on deceased people in order to ascertain the cause of death as well as the manner in which they passed away [1]. In recent years, there have been significant improvements and novel ideas in postmortem examination as a result of constant pursuit of advancement and the incorporation of cutting-edge technologies and approaches. Forensic Medicine is an application of medical knowledge for the purpose of law both civil and criminal cases [3]. The inception of forensic medicine can be historically situated in ancient civilizations. One instance of arsenic poisoning-induced homicide was recorded by the Roman statesman Cicero as early as 44 B.C. Postmortem examinations were a customary practice in ancient China, serving the purpose of ascertaining the cause of death and dispensing justice. Prominent individuals such as Sir Bernard Spilsbury and Rudolf Virchow (The father of modern pathology) played an essential role in the development of forensic medicine and pathology [4]. Forensic medicine can be divided into a number of sub branches. Forensic pathology deals with morbid anatomy, pathology of injury and different aspects of death with their medicolegal significance. Forensic odontology where the ability of dentistry is undertaken when the question of identification and interpretation of bite marks arise [5]. Forensic dentists analyse dental records and the condition of teeth to establish the identity of the deceased when other means of identification are not possible. Dental examinations can also provide information about bite marks and dental injuries that may be linked to the cause of death. A number of factors are found in the teeth that are utilised for identification purposes. Forensic anthropology, studied of bodily shape and skeletal formation in legal sense and also for the identification purposes [5]. In cases where bodies are badly decomposed or skeletal remains are all that's left, forensic anthropologists use their expertise to identify the deceased, determine age, sex, ancestry, and potential trauma or disease-related factors.

2. Relationship between forensic science and forensic medicine

Forensic science and forensic medicine are two closely related fields that share a common objective to provide expert analysis and evidence that assists in legal investigations and the administration of justice. Forensic scientists and forensic pathologists often collaborate on cases. For example, when a deceased person is found at a crime scene, forensic scientists may collect physical evidence, such as hair, fibres, or biological samples. This evidence can then be handed over to forensic pathologists who, during an autopsy, examine the body for injuries, signs of poison, or other medical conditions. This collaboration can help establish a more comprehensive understanding of the circumstances surrounding a death or a crime.

3. Role of forensic science in post-mortem examinations

Forensic science plays an important part in post-mortem investigations which are conducted on deceased individuals to determine the cause and manner of death by providing a variety of modern tools, techniques, and expertise essential to systematically gather, analyse, and examine various types of evidence [6]. Often, a prevalent inquiry arises: "What is the importance of investigating the death of an individual who is beyond assistance?" [3]. Although the deceased cannot directly profit from such a study, its importance exists in its potential to help the living and future generations [7]. It is crucial to establish the cause of death in forensic aspect that highly values the sanctity of life. During circumstances of unexpected fatal accidents, the forensic pathologist assumes a crucial position in determining the cause of death. The cooperation among forensic scientists, forensic pathologists, and medical examiners is essential in conducting these examinations, ensuring thorough examination of each case and helps in revealing the facts.

3.1 Cause of death determination

In forensic postmortem examinations, the determination of the cause of death is a critical aspect. Forensic pathologists, who are medical doctors specialised in examining deceased individuals, thoroughly investigate the body to identify the underlying condition or circumstances that led to the person's death [1]. The cause of death can fall into several broad categories, and it's essential to establish it accurately for legal and investigative purposes. Following below are common causes of death identified during forensic postmortem examinations:

1. *Natural causes*: These are deaths that result from diseases or medical conditions. Common natural causes include:

    a. Cardiovascular diseases (e.g., heart attacks, strokes)

    b. Respiratory diseases (e.g., pneumonia)

    c. Infectious diseases (e.g., sepsis)

    d. Neurological conditions (e.g., epilepsy, brain tumours)

    e. Metabolic disorders (e.g., diabetes)

2. *Trauma and injuries*: Deaths due to external physical forces or injuries are categorised as traumatic deaths [6]. Examples include:

    a. Blunt force trauma (e.g., from falls or assaults)

   b. Sharp force trauma (e.g., stabbings, gunshot wounds)

   c. Asphyxia (e.g., strangulation or suffocation)

   d. Burns or electrocution

   e. Motor vehicle accidents

3. *Toxicological causes*: These involve deaths resulting from exposure to toxic substances, drugs, or chemicals:

   a. Poisonings (e.g., overdose of drugs, exposure to toxic chemicals)

   b. Drug-related deaths (e.g., opioids, stimulants)

   c. Alcohol intoxication

4. *Asphyxiation*: Deaths related to a lack of oxygen can be due to various circumstances:

   a. Drowning

   b. Strangulation

   c. Inhalation of noxious gases

   d. Choking on foreign objects

5. *Environmental causes*: These include deaths related to environmental factors:

   a. Hypothermia or hyperthermia

   b. Lightning strikes

   c. Exposure to extreme weather conditions

6. *Infectious diseases*: In some cases, infectious diseases can lead to death, especially if they are not properly diagnosed and treated.

3.2 Manner of death

Forensic science helps establish the manner of death, which falls into five main categories: natural, accidental, suicide, homicide, or undetermined [8]. The examination involves the analysis of medical and physical evidence, as well as the consideration of circumstantial factors to determine the most likely manner of death.

a. *Natural*: A death is classified as "natural" when it results from a disease or medical condition, typically of a non-violent or non-traumatic nature [6, 7].

b. *Accidental*: Accidental deaths occur when a person dies as a result of an unintentional or unexpected event [8]. Examples of accidental deaths include motor vehicle accidents, falls, drug overdoses, electrocutions, and accidental drownings. These deaths are typically not the result of deliberate actions.

c. *Suicide*: Self-inflicted injuries or poisoning may be identified as the cause of death.

d. *Homicide*: When the postmortem examination suggests that the death was a result of someone else's actions, it is classified as a homicide.

e. *Undetermined cause*: In some cases, despite thorough examination, it may not be possible to establish a definitive cause of death. These cases may be classified as "undetermined" or "unascertained."

3.3 Toxicology

Toxicological analysis plays a vital role in postmortem examinations, helping forensic experts determine whether toxic substances or drugs contributed to a person's death [9]. Toxicological findings help establish whether substances contributed to or caused the death. It involves the testing of biological samples, such as blood and urine, to detect the presence of drugs, alcohol, poisons, or toxins.

a. *Identification of toxic substances*: Toxicological analysis helps identify the presence of toxic substances in the deceased's body, such as drugs, alcohol, prescription medications, poisons, or chemicals [9]. This is crucial for understanding whether the individual was exposed to substances that could have played a role in their death.

b. *Determining the cause of death*: In cases where toxic substances are identified, toxicological analysis helps establish whether these substances were the primary cause of death or contributed to it. For example, an overdose of a drug or alcohol poisoning may be identified as the primary cause of death.

c. *Quantifying drug levels*: Toxicological testing quantifies the concentration of substances in the body, providing information about the amount of a drug or toxin present. In cases involving accidents or fatalities, toxicological analysis can determine whether the deceased was under the influence of drugs or alcohol at the time of the incident.

d. *Identifying illicit substances*: Illicit drugs, such as opioids, cocaine, or methamphetamines, can be detected through toxicological analysis. These findings can be relevant in drug-related deaths or cases of substance abuse.

3.4 Injury analysis

In forensic postmortem examination, the analysis of injuries is a fundamental aspect of determining the cause of death and understanding the circumstances surrounding a fatality. Within the realm of law, a wound refers to a damage that disrupts the integrity of the skin [10]. Forensic pathologists and experts employ these methods to identify, document, and interpret injuries, providing a comprehensive picture of what transpired prior to death [2]. The information gleaned from injury analysis not only contributes to the pursuit of justice in homicide cases but also aids in accident investigations, suicide determinations, and the prevention of future harm, particularly in cases of child abuse.

Injury analysis begins with the identification and thorough documentation of all injuries present on the deceased's body. These can range from contusions, lacerations, abrasions, and gunshot wounds to fractures, stab wounds, burns, and more [3]. Forensic pathologists meticulously examine these injuries, noting their location, size, shape, depth, and associated characteristics to determine the type of trauma that occurred [10]. For example, the distinct patterns of bruising and fractures can help differentiate between blunt force trauma, sharp force trauma, and gunshot injuries.

It can also enable experts to estimate the force and direction of an injury, which can be vital in homicide investigations. For instance, the direction of a gunshot wound's trajectory can provide information about the position and proximity of the shooter, helping to corroborate or refute witness testimonies. The examination of injuries also includes assessing their age and healing status. This can help determine whether injuries were recent or occurred some time before death, shedding light on potential patterns of abuse, neglect, or repeated trauma.

3.5 Histopathology

Histopathological examination involves the microscopic analysis of tissue samples collected from various organs and body parts of the deceased individual including the heart, lungs, liver, kidneys, brain, and others [11]. The selection of specific tissues for examination depends on the circumstances and findings of the macroscopic autopsy. This examination provides detailed information about the condition of the tissues and organs, helps uncover underlying diseases or injuries where cause of death is unknown, and contributes to the overall determination of the cause and manner of death [12].

3.6 Entomology

Forensic entomology is a specialised branch of forensic science that leverages the study of insects to provide essential information in criminal investigations and legal matters [5]. Insects are the first responders to a corpse, and their colonisation patterns can provide crucial information about when death occurred. By identifying the types of insects present, their life stages, and environmental conditions, entomologists can make reasonably accurate estimates of the post-mortem intervals which is the time that has elapsed since a person's death, the manner of death, aiding in the pursuit of justice [13]. Forensic entomology can be utilised to determine whether the death occurred at the scene of the body's discovery or whether the body was transported after death. Specific insect species are drawn to different environments and microclimates, and their existence can provide clues about the location of death.

4. Advancements in forensic medicine

The capacities and accuracy of post-mortem examinations have been greatly improved by advancements in forensic medicine, revolutionising the area of forensic science and its uses in criminal investigations and legal proceedings. Among the noteworthy developments are given below.

4.1 Minimally invasive autopsy techniques

The area of post-mortem investigations has undergone a revolution with the advent of minimally invasive autopsy techniques, such as "Virtopsy" meaning virtual autopsies that make use of magnetic resonance imaging (MRI) and computed tomography (CT) scans [14]. In order to conduct thorough investigations without the necessity for traditional invasive autopsies, forensic pathologists can now visualise interior organs, tissues, and pathological alterations in three dimensions thanks to non-invasive imaging technologies [14]. This development improves the acceptance and accessibility of post-mortem exams by reducing the invasiveness and time needed for operations while also making it easier to preserve the body for cultural or religious reasons.

4.2 Automated histological analysis

Digitalization and automation have revolutionised post-mortem examinations by enabling quick and accurate evaluation of tissue samples and histopathological alterations. Daisuke Komura and Shumpei Ishikawa reviewed about the machine learning methods in histopathological imaging technologies to analyse disease processes, cellular structures, and tissue shape quickly and efficiently [15]. This helps to identify abnormal findings more quickly and streamlines the diagnosis process. Forensic pathologists can precisely analyse and categorise histology data by utilising sophisticated image analysis algorithms and machine learning approaches [15]. This helps with the exact identification and characterisation of various pathological diseases and cellular abnormalities.

4.3 Advanced imaging technologies

The visualisation and analysis of post-mortem specimens have been completely transformed by the incorporation of advanced imaging technologies, including multispectral imaging, three-dimensional (3D) imaging, and sophisticated microscopy techniques. In a study conducted by Shereen Ahmad et.al mentioned about the Postmortem multislice computed tomography (PMCT) technique for autopsies which is a Modern imaging technology and a non-invasive technique which provide forensic pathology experts to improved clarity and accuracy by visualising microscopic tissue structures, lesions, cellular abnormalities, and wound path visualisation in high-resolution and detail [16]. These cutting-edge imaging technologies enable forensic pathologists to perform exhaustive and comprehensive analyses, making it easier to precisely identify and document important forensic evidence and pathological findings. PMCT can be used as a post-mortem alternative or as an autopsy complement to capture multidimensional data and produce accurate anatomical reconstructions (**Figure 1**) [16].

4.4 Forensic molecular pathology

Molecular abnormalities, disease markers, and genetic mutations can now be identified through post-mortem examinations thanks to the development of forensic molecular pathology techniques such as genetic profiling and next-generation sequencing (NGS) [17]. Shahad A Alzahrani et al. reviewed to highlight the genetic

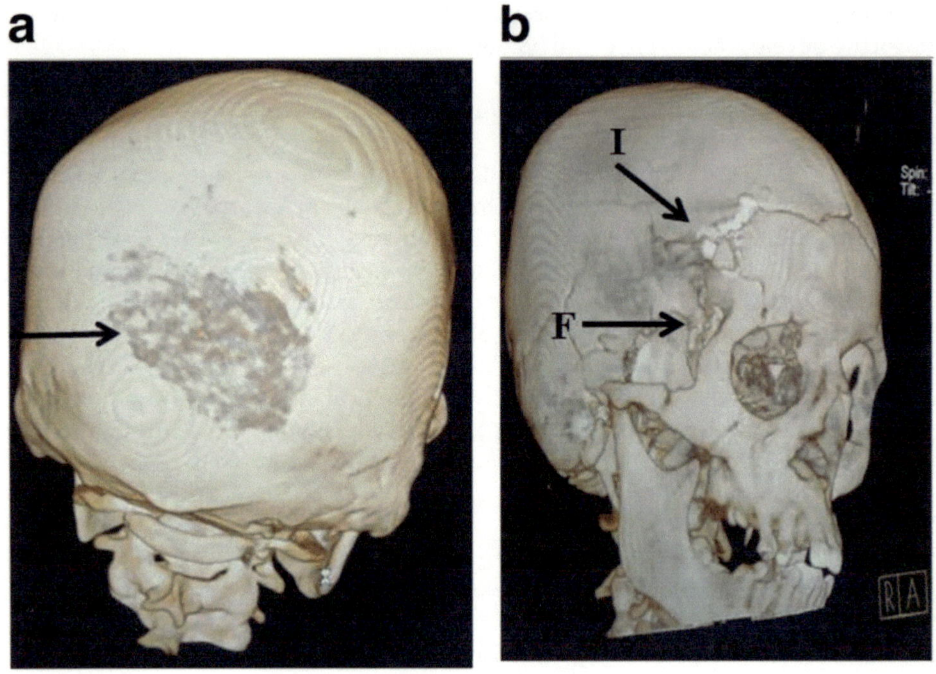

Figure 1.
Gunshot injuries of the head. A PMCT-3D-volume rendering image showing a comminuted fracture (F) opposite the exit in the occipital bone. b MDCT-3D-volume rendering image showing the entry wound of firearm injury (I) in the right temple and multiple fracture (F) of the skull bone in the right sphenoid wing, right temporal, right frontal, and right occipital bone [15].

causes of sudden death with the help of postmortem genetic testing (molecular autopsy) technique [18]. It helps forensic experts to identify genetic predispositions and familial disease risks by incorporating molecular pathology analyses into post-mortem investigations. This allows for the discovery of critical information regarding the genetic basis of pathological conditions and hereditary diseases. In the context of forensic medicine, the use of NGS technology facilitates thorough genomic analysis and the identification of particular genetic variants and mutations, which helps with the accurate diagnosis and classification of genetic and hereditary disorders. Dewar et al. undertook an investigation to determine the genetic disorders in autopsy cases by utilising postmortem genetic testing to investigate cases of sudden unexplained death (SUD) [19].

4.5 Integrated data analysis and forensic databases

Forensic databases and integrated data analysis platforms have made it easier to gather, manage, and analyse post-mortem data. This has made it possible to retrieve, compare, and interpret data for forensic investigations and research projects more quickly and efficiently. A comprehensive and interdisciplinary approach to post-mortem examinations and forensic analyses is fostered by these cutting-edge data management systems, which give forensic professionals the ability to compile and integrate a wide range of post-mortem data, including pathological findings, toxicological results, genetic profiles, and case histories. Forensic experts can carry out thorough and methodical assessments of forensic evidence by utilising advanced data analysis tools and forensic databases. This makes it easier to accurately interpret and integrate multidimensional data sets for forensic investigations and expert testimony in court cases.

4.6 Forensic virtual reality and simulation

The training and teaching of forensic pathologists, medical examiners, and investigators has been completely transformed by the advent of forensic virtual reality (VR) and simulation technologies [20]. Forensic virtual reality and simulation platforms, through the simulation of diverse post-mortem scenarios, crime scene reconstructions, and forensic analyses, provide forensic professionals with an immersive and dynamic learning environment that fosters the development of their investigative techniques, critical thinking skills, and practical skills in a controlled and simulated forensic setting [20]. In Switzerland, juries were involved in a realistic scenario where radiologists and forensic professionals utilised Virtual Reality headsets to produce postmortem imaging, imitating trauma mechanisms and crime scenes for presentation in the court [21]. The virtually reconstructed crime scene based on 3D virtual autopsy as shown in **Figure 2**.

4.7 Routine photography and its significance in post-mortem examination

In order to support the advances in post-mortem examinations, routine injury photography is a crucial component of forensic medicine. It allows for the thorough documentation, analysis, and interpretation of traumatic injuries, wound patterns, and physical trauma. By employing sophisticated photography techniques to

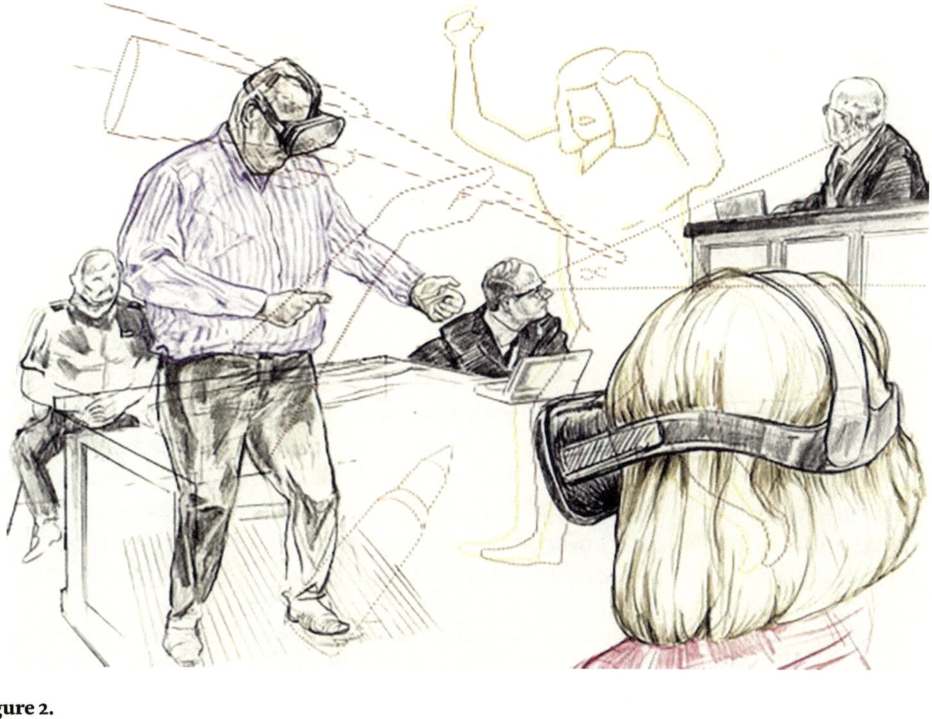

Figure 2.
3D virtual reality reconstruction of crime scene using postmortem imaging. Picture courtesy Christoph Fischer [21].

document injuries in a methodical manner, forensic experts can obtain comprehensive visual records of external trauma, anatomical alterations, and wound attributes. This allows for the accurate and dependable evaluation of injury patterns and their association with the cause and mode of death. When regular injury photography is connected to the above mentioned developments in forensic medicine, the following outcomes are seen:

a. *Comprehensive documentation and visualisation*: Traumatic injuries and anatomical changes can be comprehensively documented and visualised through the use of routine photography of injuries in conjunction with cutting-edge imaging technologies and digital visualisation tools. Through the integration of sophisticated photography techniques with multispectral imaging, three-dimensional (3D) imaging, and high-resolution microscopy, forensic experts can effectively capture precise and detailed visual depictions of injuries, improving the lucidity and accuracy of injury reports and streamlining the thorough examination and interpretation of traumatic findings in the context of post-mortem examinations.

b. *Enhanced injury analysis and pattern recognition*: The analysis and recognition of injury patterns and trauma features are improved by the combination of automated histology analysis, forensic virtual reality technologies, and routine photography. Forensic experts can perform in-depth analyses of injury patterns, wound morphology, and tissue characteristics by combining meticulous photographic records with automated image analysis algorithms and virtual reality simulations. This makes it easier to precisely identify and classify traumatic injuries and their forensic significance in the context of post-mortem investigations.

c. *Integrative data management and injury profiling*: The methodical correlation and interpretation of photographic evidence with genetic and molecular findings is made possible by routine photography of injuries combined with forensic databases and molecular pathology analyses. Forensic experts can perform multidimensional data integration and comprehensive injury profiling by integrating photographic documentation into comprehensive forensic databases and integrated data analysis platforms. This promotes an integrated approach to injury assessment and interpretation in the context of post-mortem examinations and forensic analyses.

4.8 Microbial forensics

In order to determine the origins, pathways of transmission, and potential roles of microorganisms—including bacteria, viruses, and fungi—in criminal investigations and bioterrorism incidents, forensic scientists have developed a specialised field known as "microbial forensics" [22]. Robinson et al. reviewed about the potential applications of microbiomics in forensic science which includes geolocation, personal identification, biological sex determination [23], cause and manner of death, postmortem interval investigations majorly by thanatomicrobiome [24] and trace evidence analysis by studying the presence of bacterial growth on objects and surfaces [25] as shown in **Figure 3** [26]. The following results can be shown by combining microbiological forensics with improvements in post-mortem examinations.

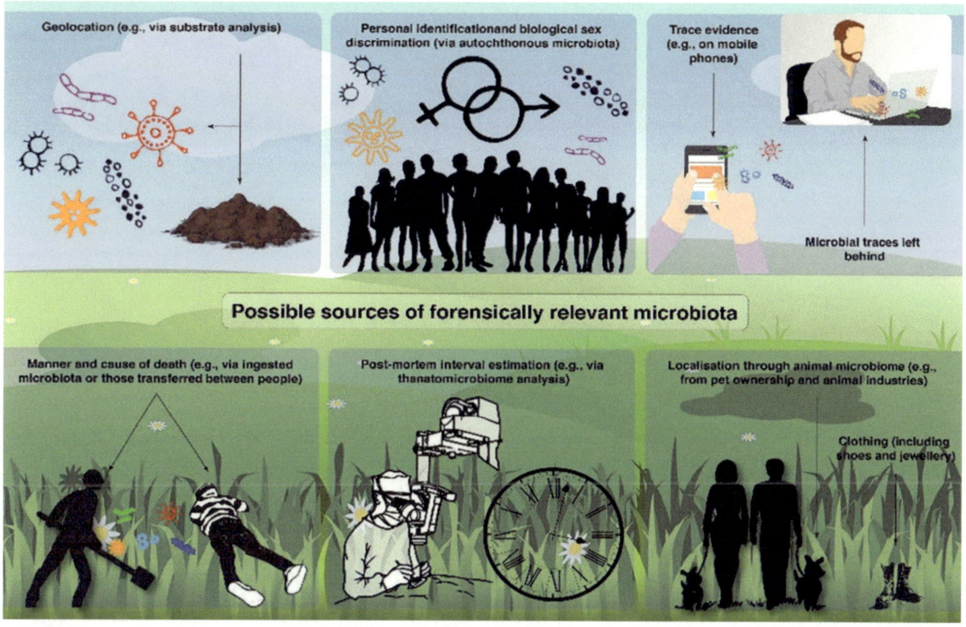

Figure 3.
Possible sources to be identified with the help of microbial forensics.

a. *Identification and profiling of pathogens and disease-causing microorganisms*: Identification and profiling of pathogens and disease-causing microorganisms linked to infectious diseases and biological threats is made possible by the integration of microbial forensics into post-mortem investigations and damage reporting [27]. Using sophisticated molecular pathology methods and microbial genomic analyses, forensic experts can pinpoint and describe particular microorganisms, making it easier to pinpoint infectious agents, their routes of transmission, and their possible roles in the onset and course of pathological conditions and disease states.

b. *Interpretation and examination of biological evidence*: Microbial forensics can be integrated with extensive data management systems and injury analysis platforms to facilitate the interpretation and analysis of microbial and biological evidence in the context of post-mortem examinations and injury. Forensic experts can perform multifaceted analyses of biological evidence by combining microbial data with extensive injury profiles and forensic databases. This allows for the integration and correlation of microbial signatures with trauma characteristics, pathological findings, and injury patterns, improving the comprehensive interpretation and forensic significance of microbial evidence in the context of criminal investigations and post-mortem analyses.

c. *Epidemiological investigations and outbreak analysis*: The conduct of epidemiological investigations and outbreak analyses of naturally occurring infectious diseases is facilitated by the integration of microbial forensics [28]. Investigators will also use the actual geographical location of the crime and evidence obtained from other forensic disciplines (e.g. PMI estimations) to reconstruct the crime and identify the persons involved [24]. This allows for the thorough assessment and documentation of microbial transmission patterns and disease dissemination pathways.

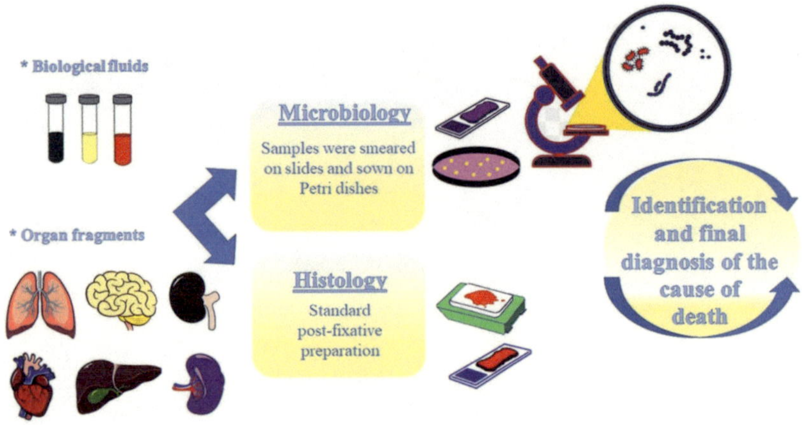

Figure 4.
Implication of the microbial forensics in post-mortem examination.

Forensic experts can examine and visualise the dynamics of disease outbreaks, the spread of infectious agents, and the connections between microbial transmission and traumatic injuries by integrating microbial data with advanced imaging modalities and injury documentation [29]. This allows for a thorough understanding of the forensic and epidemiological implications of microbial evidence in the context of post-mortem exams and injury investigations (**Figure 4**).

5. Conclusion

The utilisation of forensic science is essential to the smooth functioning of the criminal justice system. By conducting thorough analyses of evidence collected from diverse locations, such as crime scenes, forensic scientists aim to generate unbiased conclusions that aid in the investigation and legal proceedings associated with criminals, or to clear individuals who have been unfairly accused. Forensic science is especially important in the context of post-mortem examinations, also known as autopsies. Deceased individuals undergo these autopsies with the primary objective of ascertaining the cause and manner of demise. By providing the instruments and knowledge required to collect, analyse, and interpret various forms of evidence, forensic science aids medical examiners and forensic pathologists in their investigations. Integration of multiple forensic science disciplines is essential for a thorough and accurate examination of the case involving a deceased person.

Conflict of interest

The authors declare no conflict of interest.

DOI: http://dx.doi.org/10.5772/intechopen.1003870

Author details

Vaishali Abrol
National Forensic Sciences University, Gandhinagar, Gujarat, India

*Address all correspondence to: vaishaliabrol786@gmail.com

References

[1] Houck MM. Forensic Pathology. San Diego: Academic Press; 2017

[2] DiMaio VM. DiMaio's Forensic Pathology. Boca Raton: CRC Press; 2021. DOI: 10.4324/9780429318764

[3] Wagner SA. Death Scene Investigation—A Field Guide. Boca Raton: CRC Press; 2009. DOI: 10.1201/9781420086775

[4] Maude Campbell HR. The Entire History of the Autopsy. 2020. Available from: Popular Mechanics: https://www.popularmechanics.com/science/health/a25633042/autopsy-history/

[5] Amrita A. Branches of Forensic Science. 2023. Available from: Anthroholic.Com: https://anthroholic.com/branches-of-forensic-science

[6] Spitz WU. Medicolegal Investigation of Death: Guidelines for the Application of Pathology to Crime Investigation. 4th ed. Springfield, IL: Charles C. Thomas; 2006

[7] Demirci KH. Introductory chapter: An overview of post-mortem examination and autopsy. In: Dogan KH, editor. Post Mortem Examination and Autopsy – Current Issues from Death to Laboratory Analysis. Rijeka: Intech Open; 2018. p. 182

[8] Adams VI. Medicolegal autopsy and postmortem toxicology. In: Waters BL, editor. Handbook of Autopsy Practice. Totowa New Jersey: Humana Press inc; 2009. pp. 125-136

[9] Cheng WC. Postmortem toxicology: Laboratory analysis. In: Wiley Encyclopedia of Forensic Science. Hoboken, New Jersey: John Wiley and Sons; 2009

[10] Jason Payne-James RJ. Simpson's Forensic Medicine. London: Hodder & Stoughton Ltd; 2011

[11] Berney DM. Histopathology. Hoboken, New Jersey: John Wiley and Sons ltd.; 2022

[12] Siegel JA, Saukko PJ. Histopathology. In: Encyclopedia of Forensic Sciences. London, UK: Academic Press; 2013. pp. 210-216

[13] Goff ML. Forensic entomology. In: Resh VH, Cardé RT, editors. Encyclopedia of Insects. Amsterdam: Academic Press; 2009. pp. 381-386

[14] Pooja Ahuja NA. Virtopsy: A new era in forensic medico-legal autopsies. In: Dogan KH, editor. Autopsy – What Do We Learn from Corpses? Rijeka: Intech Open; 2022. DOI: 10.5772/intechopen.103781

[15] Daisuke, Komura SI. Machine learning methods for histopathological image analysis. Computational and Structural Biotechnology Journal. 2018;**16**:34-42

[16] Elkhateeb SA et al. Postmortem computed tomography and autopsy for detection of lesions and causes of death in gunshot injury cases: A comparative study. Egyptian Journal of Forensic Sciences. 2018;**8**:1-9. DOI: 10.1186/s41935-018-0078-2

[17] National Society of Genetic Counselors. (2023). Genetic profiling in post-mortem examinations. Available from: NSGC.ORG: https://www.nsgc.org/postmortem

[18] Alzahrani SA et al. Postmortem genetic testing in sudden unexpected

death: A narrative review. Cureus. 2023;**15**(1):1-9. DOI: 10.7759/cureus.33728

[19] Dewar LJ et al. Investigating the genetic causes of sudden unexpected death in children through targeted next-generation sequencing analysis. Circulation: Cardiovascular. Genetics. 2017;**10**:3-7. DOI: 10.1161/CIRCGENETICS.116.001738

[20] Bolliger SA, Thali MJ, Ross S, Buck U, Naether S, Vock P. Virtual autopsy using imaging: Bridging radiologic and forensic sciences. A review of the Virtopsy and similar projects. European Radiology. 2008;**18**(2):273-282. DOI: 10.1007/s00330-007-0737-4

[21] Monk FR. Virtual reality and postmortem imaging bring crime scenes 'to life'. 2023. Available from: Aunt Minnie Com: https://www.auntminnie.com/clinical-news/mri/article/15632913/virtual-reality-and-postmortem-imaging-bring-crime-scenes-to-life

[22] Budowle B et al. Public health. Building microbial forensics as a response to bioterrorism. Science. 2003;**301**(5641):1852-1853. DOI: 10.1126/science.1090083

[23] Bell CR. Sex-related differences in the thanatomicrobiome in postmortem heart samples using bacterial gene regions V1-2 and V4. Letters in Applied Microbiology. 2018;**67**(2):144-153. DOI: 10.1111/lam.13005

[24] Javan GT et al. The Thanatomicrobiome: A missing piece of the microbial puzzle of death. Frontiers in Microbiology. 2016;**7**(225):1-7. DOI: 10.3389/fmicb.2016.00225

[25] Koroglu MG. Comparison of keypads and touch-screen mobile phones/devices as potential risk for microbial contamination. Journal of Infection in Developing Countries. 2015;**9**(12):1308-1314. DOI: 10.3855/jidc.6171

[26] Robinson JM et al. Forensic applications of Microbiomics: A review. Frontiers in Microbiology. 2020;**11**:1-13. DOI: 10.3389/fmicb.2020.608101

[27] National Research Council. Science Needs for Microbial Forensics: Developing Initial International Research Priorities. Washington (DC): National Academies Press (US); 2014

[28] Ungria AE. Methods used in microbial forensics and epidemiological investigations for stronger health systems. Forensic Sciences Research. 2022;**7**(4):650-661. DOI: 10.1080/20961790.2021.2023272

[29] Greenwood M. News Medical Lifesciences. 2019. Available from: News-Medical.net – An AzoNetwork Site: https://www.news-medical.net/life-sciences/What-is-Microbial-Forensics.aspx